YOUR HEALTHY BODY,
YOUR HEALTHY LIFE

MasterMedia books are available at a discount with bulk purchase for educational, group, premium, or sales promotion use. For information, please write or call:

Special Sales Department
MasterMedia Limited
215 Park Avenue South
Suite 1601
New York, NY 10003
(212) 260-5600

YOUR HEALTHY BODY, YOUR HEALTHY LIFE

How to Take Control of Your Medical Destiny

Donald B. Louria, M.D.

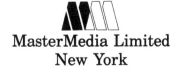

MasterMedia Limited
New York

MASTERMEDIA and colophon are registered trademarks of MasterMedia Limited.

Library of Congress Cataloging-in-Publication Data

Louria, Donald B.
Your healthy body, your healthy life: how to take control of your medical destiny/Donald B. Louria.
p.   cm.
Includes index.
ISBN 0-942361-12-1
1. Self-care, Health. 2. Medicine, Preventive. I. Title.
RA776.95.L68   1989
613—dc20   89-12151
                                CIP

Designed by Ellen Epstein for Martin Cook Associates.

Manufactured in the United States of America.

10 9 8 7 6 5 4 3 2 1

To that thoughtful man who said, "A wise person will simultaneously learn from the past, react to the present and plan for both the imminent and more distant future."

Contents

Introduction

As a young doctor, during the early years of my medical career, I devoted my time and attention to the many problems of internal medicine, infectious disease, and drug abuse. But it was not until 1969, when I was appointed chairman of the Department of Preventive Medicine and Community Health of the New Jersey Médical School, that I realized the American public was making almost no effort to prevent disease, and little effort to ensure good health and long life.

It was true then—and is true today—that most adults fall into one of four groups:

- Those who do virtually nothing to prevent disease.
- Others who spend a considerable amount of money on programs and consultations that are well advertised but inadequately documented and largely ineffective. These consumers spend too much and get too little. A well-known example: the annual executive physical examination.
- Still others who will spend outrageous sums on totally undocumented procedures offered by those who might be charlatans. Many of the megavitamin recommendations, health diets, and longevity prescriptions are included in this category.
- Finally, a small percentage of Americans who do follow sound principles of prevention. Fortunately, the number is growing.

I thought then, when I started my new assignment, that part of the problem was the failure of the preventive medicine fraternity to offer an effective program to teach healthful practices to the American public.

Any good program should be:

1

- As simple as possible.
- Well documented.
- Comprehensive.
- Easy to implement.
- Inexpensive.
- Reasonably pleasant to carry out.
- Gimmick-free.
- Cost-effective.
- Flexible, so it can be modified as new data become available.

For five years, I sifted through the available data and applied my findings to a fourteen-point Stay Well Program that was focused primarily on heart disease, cancer, and stroke. For the next four years, I crisscrossed the country talking about and refining the program, and, in 1982, it was published as a book, *Stay Well.*

In 1982, I was surprisingly naïve. I thought that all I had to do was offer to the public a sensible, well-documented program that would help them to live longer, healthier lives and everyone would immediately embrace it.

They did not, and it was clear that I would have to do more to get the message across. In 1984, Dr. Leon Smith, a colleague and friend, read the book, liked my ideas, and suggested that we make the Stay Well Program available to the public ourselves. Dr. Smith owned a small, quaint building in Roseland, New Jersey, and in the early part of 1985, we opened our first center.

Because another company had laid claim to the name "Stay Well," we had to cast about for another—one that truly reflected our message. Nothing seemed quite right.

One evening, I was sitting on my front steps with my wife, Barbara, and my seventeen-year-old daughter, Anne, as we all desperately tried to think of an appropriate name for our program. Anne suggested "healthful life." I thought about it, wrote it down, and said, "Too dull. It just doesn't say what we want to tell people." As I got up to go into the house, she said, "Dad, two words."

It was perfect. The Health-Full-Life Program says exactly what we want to say—full of life, full of health. Our logo shows a scale balancing an ounce of prevention and a pound of cure. The scale is tipped in favor of the ounce of prevention, illustrating our motto: "Tip the scales in your favor."

I am convinced the Health-Full-Life Program is the best there is. It fulfills all nine criteria for an effective program discussed earlier. I believe that if you follow our seventeen-point program, you potentially add years to your life.

1

The
Health-Full-Life
Program

The Health-Full-Life Program contains the most important elements necessary for a healthy life. The seventeen recommendations are the basics—the bedrock of any prevention program (see table 1).

Before we discuss the details of our program, it is important that the reader understand exactly what I mean when I talk about the different stages of prevention, as the whole point of my efforts is to aid the public in preventing disease before it gains a foothold and becomes a problem that must be treated.

Primary Prevention

Primary prevention is the ideal—the prevention of disease by modification of risk factors or by alteration of the individual's resistance. A risk factor is anything that promotes the occurrence of a disease. Cigarette smoking is the major risk factor for lung cancer. If you don't smoke, your chances of developing the most common form of lung cancer are virtually nil; if your reason for not smoking is to avoid lung cancer, that is avoidance of a risk factor and is primary prevention. If it were possible to remove the cancer-causing elements in cigarettes, this would be modification of the risk factor (cigarette tobacco) and would also be a form of primary prevention. In a sense, that is what low-tar, low-nicotine, filtered cigarettes are trying (with some success) to do. Immu-

TABLE 1

The Health-Full-Life Program

Test or Action	Age at Start and Frequency
1. Blood pressure determination	Yearly after age twenty
2. Blood cholesterol level	Yearly after age twenty
3. Blood high-density protein (HDL) level	Yearly after age twenty
4. Pap smear	Every two years starting at age twenty
5. Breast self-examination	Monthly starting at age thirty
6. Mammogram	Yearly starting at age forty
7. Testicular self-examination	Monthly after age twenty
8. Stool examination for presence of blood	Yearly starting at age forty
9. Blood hemoglobin determination (a test for anemia)	Yearly after age twenty
10. Left-sided bowel examination for potentially cancerous polyps	Every five years after age forty-five
11. Glaucoma eye test	Every five years after age thirty-five
12. Weight determination	Monthly
13. Immunization update	All ages
14. Daily low back exercises	Daily after age twenty
15. Smoking control	All ages
16. Nutrition and diet recommendations (adequate intake of calcium, fiber, cruciferous vegetables, and carotenes)	Always
17. Seat belt use	Always

nization to protect against polio or measles increases the individual's resistance against these viruses and is a form of primary prevention. In the long run, primary prevention is the least costly and the most effective form of prevention. Yet, it is the hardest to accomplish because ostensibly healthy people must take preventive actions *prior* to any evidence of illness.

Secondary Prevention

Secondary prevention is, in essence, early intervention. When a woman has a Pap smear taken, the physician is looking for atypical cells or completely localized cancer (so-called cancer in situ). Such cellular abnormalities and localized cancers usually remain confined to the tip of the cervix for many years before becoming invasive. If the atypical cells or cancers in situ are detected early and removed by a simple, almost painless procedure, invasive cervical cancer can be prevented. Another example of secondary prevention is detection of high blood pressure in its asymptomatic stages, when the individual feels perfectly well. If high blood pressure is detected at that point and brought under control by diet or medications, the medical consequences of high blood pressure—which include stroke, heart attacks, and kidney failure—can be avoided.

Secondary prevention, then, involves detecting sickness in its very earliest stages before there are symptoms or signs of full-blown disease and, by early treatment, preventing the disease from exerting its deleterious effects. Alternatively, the disease may be detected when minor symptoms are present but before it is fully established. For example, a man may have a chronic cough from cigarette smoking but not be otherwise ill. The cough is not only an annoyance, but also an early manifestation of chronic bronchitis, a potentially serious and life-threatening disease of the lungs. If the individual stops smoking at that point, he is practicing secondary prevention, by intervening at the earliest stages before the condition becomes severe.

Secondary prevention is, for the most part, more expensive than primary prevention, and it is not as effective because early detection fails in some cases, whereas primary prevention is often virtually completely effective.

Tertiary Prevention

Tertiary prevention is the treatment of established disease to prevent relapse or further deterioration. If a person has a heart attack, is hospitalized, and recovers from the episode, tertiary prevention would be the prevention of another heart attack. This might be done by a program of graduated exercise in some cases, by reduction in weight in others. If a blood test shows elevated cholesterol in a person who just had a heart attack, the level may be lowered by diet or medications; this is another attempt at tertiary prevention. If an individual suffers a stroke and is partially paralyzed, then tertiary prevention would involve the kind of physical rehabilitation that would prevent the initial paralysis from becoming worse.

Tertiary prevention is enormously expensive. The cost of preventing deterioration after a disease has occurred includes the cost of the disease itself, plus the accompanying efforts at rehabilitation and avoidance of relapse.

Although it is easy to say that primary prevention is less expensive than tertiary prevention, the reality is complicated. Primary prevention focuses on a whole population, whereas tertiary prevention only applies to those who get the disease. Suppose that out of 1 million adults, 400 will experience a heart attack in a given year and tertiary prevention undertaken after a heart attack would cost $10,000 per person. The total cost for that 1 million persons is 400 × $10,000, or $4 million. If it costs $10 a year for primary prevention for each person in that population, the cost for that same 1 million people would be $10 million. That would not be cost-effective. If, on the other hand, the cost of primary prevention was $5 a year, and there were expected to be 1,000 heart attacks a year in that population of 1 million people, then the cost of primary prevention would be $5 million and the cost of tertiary prevention would be $10 million; primary prevention would then be cost-effective. I have oversimplified, but the point I wish to stress is valid: primary prevention must be kept inexpensive, otherwise, it will not be cost-effective and health insurance carriers will have no incentive to support its widespread use.

Thirty percent of us will die between ages forty-five and seventy; a large percentage of those deaths can be avoided. If each adult would follow the simple program outlined in this book, a great deal of illness, hospitalization, disability, and death would be avoided or postponed for many years. That is a big payoff for the little effort required to follow the Health-Full-Life Program. (See sample health calendars for women and men on pages 9 and 10.) We don't have all the answers, but we know enough to enable you to live a longer, healthier life. You have to make the effort. This program will help you take charge of your own health.

Heart Disease

Arteriosclerotic heart disease, or hardening of the coronary arteries, is still the leading cause of death in the United States. Potentially lethal consequences of hardening of the coronary arteries are sudden death, myocardial infarction, and heart failure. A myocardial infarction is a heart attack due to loss of blood supply to the heart muscle from narrowing of the heart's blood vessels, with resulting death of some of the heart muscle. Reduction in blood supply to the heart muscle may also cause angina—chest pain around the heart area that ordinarily occurs after exertion. Angina can presage a full-blown heart attack.

In the past few decades, there has been a remarkable drop in deaths from heart attacks and coronary heart disease. The explanation for the extraordinary 40 percent reduction in deaths due to coronary heart disease is probably due to a combination of modification of risk factors and more effective

Sample Health Calendar for Women

	1989	1990	1991	1992	1993	1994	1995	1996	1997	1998
Cholesterol — MONTH DONE / RESULT — every year										
High-density lipoproteins — every year										
Blood pressure — every year										
Hemoglobin — every year										
Blood glucose (sugar) — every year										
Stools for blood yearly — MONTH DONE — after age forty										
Colon exam every five years — after age forty-five										
Glaucoma testing every five years — after age thirty-five										
Pap smear every two years — after age twenty-five										
Mammogram yearly — after age forty										
Weight—First quarter										
—Second quarter										
—Third quarter										
—Fourth quarter										

Low back exercises every day. Starting at age thirty, breast self-examination every one to three months. (Cigarettes none, or at most less than ten a day. No smoking during pregnancy. Seat belts and locked car doors—always.)

Sample Health Calendar for Men

	1989	1990	1991	1992	1993	1994	1995	1996	1997	1998
Cholesterol MONTH DONE / RESULT every two years										
High-density lipoproteins every two years										
Blood pressure every two years										
Hemoglobin every two years										
Blood glucose (sugar) every year										
Stools for blood yearly MONTH DONE after age forty										
Colon exam every five years after age forty-five										
Glaucoma testing every five years after age thirty-five										
Weight—First quarter —Second quarter —Third quarter —Fourth quarter										

Low back exercises every day. Intermittent self-examination for testicular lumps.
(Cigarettes none, or at most less than ten a day. Seat belts and locked car doors—always.)

treatment once a heart attack has occurred. Despite this fall in death rates, there are still about 600,000 deaths a year from coronary heart disease and about 1,250,000 acute heart attacks, costing more than $25 billion each year.

There are five risk factors that can be modified that are well-documented risk factors for coronary heart disease and heart attacks.

Cholesterol Level Cholesterol is a blood fat, in part derived from the diet, that can clog blood vessels. Consequently, an elevated cholesterol (over 210–220) is a major risk factor for coronary heart disease and heart attacks. Although there is still controversy about the relationship between cholesterol and heart attacks, this issue has been virtually settled by the recently completed Lipid Research Clinics Coronary Primary Prevention Trial study, summarized in the *Journal of the American Medical Association* of January 20, 1984. This study of 3,606 men with high cholesterol levels showed that reduction in cholesterol markedly reduced the risk of heart attacks; for every reduction in cholesterol of 1 percent, there was a 2 percent decrease in heart attacks. The evidence is incontestable: cholesterol levels bear a direct relationship to the likelihood of a heart attack.

In the United States, the cholesterol levels for the nation as a whole are much higher than those found in many other areas of the world. In addition, our definition of "normal" is higher than what is considered "normal" in other countries, particularly those that are less developed. Since heart attack risk is related to cholesterol level, those we define in the United States as having a high cholesterol (compared with our average or "normal") are at very considerable risk of heart attack. And, since our average or "normal" is itself relatively high, even those with "normal" cholesterol levels in this country are at some risk. Only those with levels substantially *below* normal are really at low risk.

Is there a level of cholesterol that is absolutely safe? The answer is yes, probably at around 150 milligrams, but that is a very low level, and one that is not usually found in the majority of Americans.

A National Institutes of Health panel of twenty-two experts, chaired by Dr. Dewitt Goodman of Columbia University, concluded in an October 1987 report that adults should have their blood cholesterol monitored regularly, that the goal should be a cholesterol level of 200 or less, and that those with levels over 240 should have additional tests carried out to decide whether treatment should be initiated with diet and possibly with cholesterol-lowering drugs. Those with intermediate levels (200–239) should also be retested with more detailed analyses if they have other risk factors for coronary heart disease.

An impressive study that appeared in the November 28, 1986, issue of the *Journal of the American Medical Association,* by Dr. Jeremiah Stamler and his colleagues, examined deaths among 356,222 men screened for the Multiple Risk Factor Intervention Trial. They found that any elevation of cholesterol above 180 milligrams increased the risk of death from coronary heart disease. Between 182 and 202, the increased risk was very slight, but between 203 and 220, the increase was somewhat more impressive (about 70 percent). The major increases occurred at levels over 221, particularly over 245, where more than half the excess deaths were found. Only about 10 percent of the excess deaths occurred in the 203 to 220 category. The study makes it clear that even modest levels of cholesterol carry some risk. The goal of the U.S. Department of Health and Human Services is 200 milligrams average cholesterol by 1990. That would be ideal, but for a lot of people, 200 is not realistic. Under age forty, a level of 200 is a sensible goal; for those over forty, 210 is reasonable.

In the Health-Full-Life Program, the cholesterol level in the blood is measured yearly after age twenty.

One problem with single determinations of cholesterol is the accuracy of the laboratory test. The April 24, 1987, issue of *The Medical Letter* reported the results of a study by the American College of Pathologists in which a large number of laboratories were sent blood samples and asked to determine the cholesterol level. The results were discouraging; the range of results from reputable laboratories on a single specimen with known cholesterol level was extraordinary. Since cholesterol results differ so much from laboratory to laboratory, or even within the same laboratory on repeated tests, it is important for each person to establish his or her own patterns and ranges by obtaining yearly cholesterol levels starting at age twenty. If a single test shows substantial elevation in the cholesterol level (greater than 240), the first step is to obtain another determination. If a single test shows moderate abnormality (up to 240), no precipitous action is necessary; moderate weight loss and a repeat test a year later is all that is required.

High-Density Lipoproteins High-density proteins combine with cholesterol and carry it away from the heart and blood vessels to be excreted. This is a somewhat simplistic explanation, but it seems clear from a variety of studies that the higher the HDL, the better, and the lower the risk of coronary heart disease and heart attacks. In this case, opposites are desirable: the lower the cholesterol, the better; the higher the HDL, the better.

If the HDL is below 40 milligrams, this is considered undesirable and such persons are more at risk of a heart attack. A level of 40–54 is considered in the average range, and over 55 milligrams is considered very good. If your level is over 45, you are less susceptible to heart attack than the person with an HDL level of 35. Women generally have much more of the protective high-density protein cholesterol and this appears to be the best explanation for the observation that they are less likely to experience coronary heart disease.

The HDL level in the blood should be measured every year and it is also useful to determine the interrelationship between cholesterol and HDL by determining the cholesterol:HDL ratio, which is thought to be of predictive value in coronary heart disease. The lower the cholesterol and the higher the HDL, the better it is. As the cholesterol falls and the HDL increases, the ratio will fall. A lower ratio signifies a lower heart disease risk. A ratio of 6 is too high, 5 is satisfactory but borderline high, 4½ is very satisfactory and 4 or less is excellent.

Blood Pressure Elevation It is absolutely clear that there is a direct relationship between the height of the blood pressure and the likelihood of developing coronary heart disease or experiencing a heart attack. There are two components to blood pressure, the higher systolic reading and the lower diastolic reading. The systolic pressure—the higher value—is the result of the thrust of the blood against the blood vessels as the heart muscle contracts and forces the blood out of the heart into the adjacent vessels. The systolic pressure should not exceed 150 in persons under age fifty and should not exceed 160 in persons over that age. (It is well to remember that as one grows older, the reading for the systolic part of the blood pressure may be somewhat higher.) When the heart relaxes between beats, the blood vessels recoil from the initial thrust of blood from the heart and that results in the diastolic pressure. It should be less than 90 at any age.

If the pressure is elevated, a repeat determination should be made the same day after a period of relaxation. If the pressure is still elevated, it should be retested on a different day after a period of sitting quietly. If it remains elevated, then the physician should decide whether treatment is necessary.

I must stress the importance of repeating blood pressure measurements if the reading is borderline high or high. The anxiety of an examination can elevate the blood pressure and it still may be elevated even if the person relaxes for fifteen minutes before retesting. Between one-fifth and one-third of those who have elevated pressure at one observation will be found to have normal blood pressure on subsequent readings.

Some people recommend determining the pressure several times a year, but there really is no good reason for doing this in a person who feels well. If the blood pressure rises precipitously between measurements, and remains markedly elevated, and this elevation poses a threat to the individual because of the rapid increase, then almost always there will be symptoms such as severe headache or shortness of breath. In the overwhelming majority of cases, the blood pressure increase will occur more gradually and detection by obtaining a blood pressure reading every year will allow plenty of time for effective intervention by diet, salt restriction, or, if necessary, medications.

Smoking Cigarette smoking is thought to account for about 20 percent of the risk for coronary heart disease and heart attacks, almost all of that among those smoking more than a half pack a day or with multiple risk factors such as high cholesterol plus smoking. If you have never smoked more than a half pack per day, in the absence of other risk factors, that amount of smoking causes only a small risk of coronary heart disease.

Although I do not believe there is convincing evidence that smoking less than a half pack a day is likely to contribute significantly to the development of a first major coronary event, any smoking may be harmful to those who have already had such an event; this would include those suffering from established coronary heart disease, heart failure, a heart attack, or angina (pain in the chest usually with exercise, sometimes even without exercise, due to a reduced blood supply to the heart muscle).

It has been suggested that filter cigarettes may actually increase the frequency of heart attacks. This has now been studied carefully by the late Cuyler Hammond, Ph.D., of the American Cancer Society. He and his colleagues have followed on a long-term basis hundreds of thousands of smokers and nonsmokers. Their report and other studies have resulted in general agreement that filter cigarettes neither increase nor decrease the likelihood of heart attacks compared with nonfilter cigarettes.

I know that my statement that less than a half pack a day is probably of little risk to the person who has no evidence of heart disease is controversial. However, it is supported by a variety of studies, including one by Lynn Rosenberg and associates published November 25, 1983, in the *Journal of the American Medical Association.* They studied 255 women who had had a heart attack when they were not yet fifty years of age. Smoking was a major risk factor for those who smoked fifteen or more cigarettes per day, but it was not a risk factor at all for those smoking less than a half pack a day.

Beneficial effects begin reasonably soon after smoking is discontinued. How long after a one- or two-pack-a-day smoker stops does the excess risk related to smoking completely disappear? According to a study by Lynn Rosenberg and her colleagues, presented at the annual meeting of the Society for Epidemiologic Research in North Carolina in June 1985, the answer is about two years. Others have said one year, but on the basis of the present evidence, I think two years is the most sensible time frame to use. If you have smoked more, say one to two packs a day, and reduce that amount to less than a half pack per day, will the risk of coronary heart disease or lung cancer fall to that of a person who never smoked more than a half pack per day? No one really knows the answer. That is one good reason for the moderately heavy to heavy smoker (one pack per day or more) to stop altogether rather than reduce the number of cigarettes to less than a half pack per day.

There is one group for which half a pack a day or less for healthy persons should not apply: pregnant women. The most important cause of death in the first month of life is low birth weight of the infant (defined as less than five and a half pounds). It has been shown by many investigators that the size of the baby is related to the smoking history of the mother during pregnancy; the likelihood of having a low-birth-weight baby is much greater if the mother smokes regularly.

Is this effect on the growth of the baby during pregnancy dose-related? Absolutely. The weight is directly correlated with the amount smoked. If a woman is pregnant, it would be best if she smoked not at all or only occasionally. If she does smoke, she must limit herself to one to three cigarettes a day if she cares for her unborn child. If she does not limit herself, especially if she smokes more than a half pack daily, she is not showing proper concern for her baby; that baby is more likely to develop inadequately, to weigh less than five and a half pounds at birth, and as a result to be at greater risk of death during the first month of life.

Another group of persons who should not smoke at all are those with chronic bronchitis. Bronchitis is an inflammatory disease of the bronchial tubes leading from the mouth to the lungs. It is characterized by cough and the production of sputum. Acute bronchitis is usually due to viruses or bacteria and lasts from a few days to two to three weeks. There is no way of preventing acute bronchitis.

The chronic form of bronchitis is a different story. It occurs almost exclusively as a consequence of cigarette smoking. It starts with a cough and with the production of a little sputum, usually in the morning right after the individual awakens. This is the first phase. The second stage is the occurrence of intermittent infections due to a variety of organisms. The third stage results both from damage to the lungs caused by the infections and that inflicted by the initial cause of this disease, tobacco smoke. At this stage, the victim coughs a great deal, brings up a lot of phlegm, is short of breath, often wheezes, and suffers many infections. The lungs are then abnormally distended and the disease is called chronic bronchitis with emphysema. Anyone with chronic bronchitis must not smoke at all.

There is some risk from any cigarette smoking and abstinence is surely the best policy, but if you have to smoke, less than a half pack a day is the cut-off point between minimal danger and considerable danger. If you have a high cholesterol level, a low HDL level, or high blood pressure, you should not be smoking at all.

When my first book on prevention, *Stay Well*, was published in 1982, many people criticized the recommendations on smoking. They did not quarrel with my facts, but they felt that most smokers would not limit themselves to a half pack a day or less and that we should condemn any smoking. I countered by noting that one-quarter of smokers did limit themselves to a half pack a day or less and I believed many more would do so with proper education. Besides, I thought we must stick strictly to the facts.

The facts in 1989 are no different, but I want to emphasize very strongly that limiting the number of cigarettes to less than a half pack a day is clearly second best. I urge strongly that everybody should avoid or stop cigarette smoking. And it all goes back to Rachel Carson's *Silent Spring,* that seminal and marvelous book, written in 1962. In emphasizing the potentially catastrophic effects of a hodgepodge of chemicals we were spewing into our environment, she kept stressing the dangers of unknown long-term effects of exposure to multiple chemicals in various combinations. She said,

> Within the groups of chemicals themselves there are sinister and little understood, interacting transformations and summations of effects . . . this piling up of chemicals from many different sources creates a total exposure that cannot be measured. . . . Chemicals sprayed on croplands or forests or gardens pass mysteriously by underground streams until they emerge and through the alchemy of air and sunlight combine into new forms that kill vegetation, sicken cattle and work unknown harm on those who drink from once pure wells.

Those concerns are even more true today, and they apply directly to cigarette smoking. We are all exposed to multiple toxins every day. Some we ingest with our food and water; others are inhaled and are potentially dangerous to the lungs. We may breathe in a little asbestos, some radon from our homes, and a tiny amount of long-lasting radioactivity from Chernobyl (or radioactive materials released from our nuclear weapons factories or from accidental releases such as that at Three Mile Island). And then, there may be indoor pollution in some homes from substances such as formaldehyde. Each of these may be inhaled in small amounts, so the regulators and scientists are able to tell us that the concentration of what we inhaled was below the danger level. But who will assure us that multiple toxic substances inhaled together will not induce long-term effects when acting together?

The long-term effects of chemicals and radioactive substances acting in concert could be various kinds of lung damage, or lung cancer. That being true, why add to the potential lung insult by smoking tobacco? We know that among those exposed to asbestos or uranium, the likelihood of lung cancer is markedly increased among those who also smoke cigarettes. If you take a little bit of asbestos, a little bit of radon, a little bit of radioactive substance, a little bit of all sorts of other toxins, adding even a little bit of cigarette smoke may increase the potential for lung damage or perhaps even heart disease.

Think about Rachel Carson's prescient warnings: if you must smoke, less than a half pack a day of the low-tar, filtered type should be your daily limit. Not smoking at all is much, much better.

Overweight Is overweight a risk factor for coronary heart disease and heart attacks by itself? The answer is yes, but by itself it is the least important of the five major risk factors related to heart disease.

There are several issues of importance. One is that the definition of overweight changes with time and with the age of the individual. There is no agreement on the dividing line between normal and excessive weight for either men or women. Another problem is that many of the best studies divide the subjects into those less than 10 percent overweight, between 10 and 29 percent overweight, and more than 30 percent overweight. That makes it difficult to tell where the danger point exists in the middle group. It could be at 15 or 20 or 25 percent above the ideal. At the time I wrote *Stay Well,* almost everyone used the Metropolitan Life figures for each age group according to sex and body frame (small, medium, or large). These figures were altered in 1983 (see table 2) to permit a few extra pounds in each group.

In February 1985, a National Institutes of Health panel

TABLE 2

1983 Metropolitan Life Insurance Company Height and Weight Chart

MEN

Height	Small Frame	Medium Frame	Large Frame
5' 1"	123–129	126–136	133–145
5' 2"	125–131	128–138	135–148
5' 3"	127–133	130–140	137–151
5' 4"	129–135	132–143	139–155
5' 5"	131–137	134–146	141–159
5' 6"	133–140	137–149	144–163
5' 7"	135–143	140–152	147–167
5' 8"	137–146	143–155	150–171
5' 9"	139–149	146–158	153–175
5'10"	141–152	149–161	156–179
5'11"	144–155	152–165	159–183
6' 0"	147–159	155–169	163–187
6' 1"	150–163	159–173	167–192
6' 2"	153–167	162–177	171–197
6' 3"	157–171	166–182	176–202

WOMEN

Height	Small Frame	Medium Frame	Large Frame
4' 9"	99–108	106–116	115–129
4'10"	100–110	108–120	117–131
4'11"	101–112	110–123	119–134
5' 0"	103–115	112–126	122–137
5' 1"	105–118	115–129	125–140
5' 2"	108–121	118–132	128–144
5' 3"	111–124	121–135	131–148
5' 4"	114–127	124–138	134–152
5' 5"	117–130	127–141	137–156
5' 6"	120–133	130–144	140–160
5' 7"	123–136	133–147	143–164
5' 8"	126–139	136–150	146–167
5' 9"	129–142	139–153	149–170
5'10"	132–145	142–156	152–173
5'11"	135–148	145–159	155–176

NOTE: The chart has been adjusted so that figures apply to weight and height determined without clothes or shoes.

defined obesity as being about four to five pounds heavier for women than the maximum allowed in the Metropolitan Life charts and eight to nine pounds heavier for men. Another very well-respected unit, the Gerontology Research Center, allows much more weight gain in the middle years (see table 3).

Clearly, the experts disagree about exactly what the ideal weight should be for a given person.

Another unsettled issue is the best measurement of obesity. The most frequently used is weight for a given height, sex, and body build. That is the basis for the Metropolitan Life charts. More sophisticated and arguably better is the body-mass index, defined as the weight divided by the square of the height. To complicate matters, there is growing enthusiasm for a new measurement called "abdominal obesity." This is a ratio of the circumference at the midabdomen divided by the circumference at the hips. Those with flat tummies do well; those with pot bellies do not.

There are two important questions concerning the usefulness of abdominal obesity in predicting the initial occurrence or the later recurrence of heart attacks or strokes. The first is whether measurement of abdominal obesity adds to information gained from other measurements of weight (such as weight:height ratios). The answer is probably yes. The second question is whether the ratio of abdominal girth to hip girth is more useful than other measurements and is predictive of occurrence of heart attack or stroke even if other, older measurements fall within the normal range. The answer, at least in regard to stroke and heart attacks, is not yet known.

Will being 10 percent overweight in itself cause heart disease? The answer is no.

What if you are from 11 to 20 percent overweight? That would mean a 120-pound woman at ideal weight could weigh up to 144 pounds and the 160-pound man at ideal weight could weigh up to 192 pounds. That is a fair amount of excess baggage to carry. Yet, the available evidence suggests that the likelihood of heart disease is not significantly increased.

It is clear that the more weight you gain above the ideal

TABLE 3

Gerontology Research Center:
Age-Specific Weight Range for Men and Women

Height (feet and inches)	Weight (age 20–29)	Weight (age 30–39)	Weight (age 40–49)	Weight (age 50–59)	Weight (age 60–69)
4′10″	84–111	92–119	99–127	107–135	115–142
4′11″	87–115	95–123	102–131	111–139	119–147
5′ 0″	90–119	98–127	106–135	114–143	123–152
5′ 1″	93–123	101–131	110–140	118–148	127–157
5′ 2″	96–127	105–136	113–144	122–153	131–163
5′ 3″	99–131	108–140	117–149	126–158	135–168
5′ 4″	102–135	112–145	121–154	130–163	140–173
5′ 5″	106–140	115–149	125–159	134–168	144–179
5′ 6″	109–144	119–154	129–164	138–174	148–184
5′ 7″	112–148	122–159	133–169	143–179	153–190
5′ 8″	116–153	126–163	137–174	147–184	158–196
5′ 9″	119–157	130–168	141–179	151–190	162–201
5′10″	122–162	134–173	145–184	156–195	167–207
5′11″	126–167	137–178	149–190	160–201	172–213
6′ 0″	129–171	141–183	153–195	165–207	177–219
6′ 1″	133–176	145–188	157–200	169–213	182–225
6′ 2″	137–181	149–194	162–206	174–219	187–232
6′ 3″	141–186	153–199	166–212	179–225	192–238
6′ 4″	144–191	157–205	171–218	184–231	197–244

level, the more likely it is that your cholesterol, blood sugar, and blood pressure levels will increase to abnormal levels and that your high-density protein (HDL) levels will fall.

I would emphasize that not all cholesterol or blood pressure or blood sugar elevations are related to weight, and in many instances they will persist even after significant weight loss.

The cut-off point for dangerously excessive weight is 20 to 30 percent above ideal weight. In some studies, such as the famous Framingham, Massachusetts, long-term study of risk factors for coronary heart disease, the cut-off point was primarily at 30 percent overweight; in other studies, it has been 20 percent. A prudent view of overweight would set the danger point at 20 percent, even taking into account the individual variations based on bone and muscle structure. At that amount of overweight, there is even greater likelihood of abnormalities of cholesterol, high-density lipoproteins, blood pressure, and blood sugar.

Although this degree of overweight is a risk factor by itself (independent of cholesterol or blood pressure) for coronary heart disease, it is a minor risk factor. For heart disease, cholesterol elevation and high blood pressure, as well as smoking, are more important risk factors.

Of course, once the critical cut-off point for dangerous increase in weight is reached, the more excessive the weight, the greater the risk. Forty percent overweight is a lot more dangerous than 25 percent overweight.

How, then, do you calculate 20 percent overweight? From the midpoint of each range in the Metropolitan Life and Gerontology Research Center range? From the upper level of "normal"? If the experts can't agree on the definition of normal weight, what are we supposed to do or think?

In view of the somewhat divergent data, Health-Full-Life has adopted a commonsense compromise. For those under age forty, we will define potentially dangerous overweight as 20 percent above the *midpoint* of the "normal" range for their sex, height, and frame according to the 1983 Metropolitan Life table. For those over age forty, we will permit somewhat greater weight gain; we will define potentially dangerous weight gain at 20 percent above the *upper limit* of the "normal" range for their sex, height, and frame. That 20 percent is still a lot of leeway. A man with a large frame who should weight 180 pounds can actually weigh 216 pounds before reaching the danger point.

One question often asked is what percentage of those persons who suffer heart attacks have no obvious abnormalities in risk factors. The answer is perhaps one-third of the time. Part of that one-third is genetic, that is, inherited. But part relates to the fact that cholesterol and blood pressure measurement are each on a continuum. Cholesterol of 220 is considered, at worst, borderline elevated, but that is well above the no-risk cholesterol level, and a person with a cholesterol of 220 is more at risk for a heart attack than a person with a cholesterol of 190. Similarly, a person with a blood pressure of 110/60 is at lesser risk of heart attack than a person with a blood pressure of 139/85, even though both are in the normal range. So you cannot be complacent just because your values are in the "normal" range. The closer you get to the ideal, the better it is for your health.

I would recommend some action for anyone with a cholesterol level of over 210 at any age, or an HDL of less than 40, or a cholesterol:HDL ratio of over 4½. A recent estimate suggests that 60 million American adults need to lower their cholesterol levels. I would also recommend some corrective measures for any person under fifty years of age with a blood pressure greater than 148/88, or for a person over fifty years of age with blood pressure above 158/88.

What actions should be taken if the cholesterol is elevated or the HDL is too low or the blood pressure is too high? The sequential actions are listed in table 4. Note that if the cholesterol is elevated and the individual is overweight or even in the upper half of the normal weight range for his or her age, the treatment is weight loss. If the individual is low-normal weight or underweight, a low-cholesterol, low-saturated-fat diet is recommended with a commensurate increase in use of unsaturated fats. The evidence for a low-cholesterol, low-fat diet lowering cholesterol levels, even in the absence of weight loss, is impressive. For example, a study by Christian Ehnholm and his colleagues published in the *New England Journal of Medicine* of September 30, 1982, showed that the cholesterol level could be predicted by diet; on a diet with a lot of fatty meat, cheese, butter, and milk, it was high; but if a

TABLE 4

Health-Full-Life Approach to Moderately Elevated Cholesterol, Moderately Elevated Blood Pressure, Low High-Density Lipoprotein Levels

If Person Is	Moderately High Cholesterol	Moderately Elevated Blood Pressure	Low Levels of High-Density Lipoproteins (HDL)
Overweight	1. Weight-loss diet. 2. Add exercise, if needed. 3. Add low-cholesterol, low-fat diet, if needed.	1. Weight-loss diet. 2. Add exercise, if needed. 3. Add salt restriction, if needed. 4. If 1, 2, and 3 fail, consider antihypertensive drugs.*	1. Weight-loss diet and stop smoking. 2. If needed, add exercise. 3. Can also consider two alcoholic drinks a day.
Normal weight	1. Weight-loss diet and exercise. 2. Add low-cholesterol, low-fat diet, if needed.	1. Weight-loss diet and exercise. 2. Add salt restriction, if needed. 3. If 1 and 2 fail, consider antihypertensive drugs.*	1. Weight-loss diet and stop smoking. 2. If needed, add exercise. 3. Can also consider two alcoholic drinks a day.
Below normal weight	1. Low-fat, low-cholesterol diet. 2. Add exercise, if needed.	1. Exercise. 2. If needed, add salt restriction. 3. If 1 and 2 fail, consider antihypertensive drugs.*	1. Exercise and stop smoking. 2. Can also consider taking one to two alcoholic drinks a day (but no more than that).

*Prior to using drugs, stress reduction may be tried.

skimmed-milk, lean-meat, low-fat-cheese diet using margarine and lots of poultry was substituted, the cholesterol level fell markedly.

There are many other studies that agree with Ehnholm's. If a person who should be able to lose weight does not by diet alone, then an exercise program is recommended as a help in losing weight. If weight loss is achieved but it does not help in lowering the cholesterol, then that person is placed on the low-cholesterol, low-fat diet.

If the individual who is low-normal weight or underweight achieves inadequate cholesterol reduction on a low-fat, low-cholesterol diet, an exercise program is added. There is some as yet inconclusive evidence that some cholesterol reduction will occur with exercise in the absence of weight loss.

To sum up: You can lower cholesterol by reducing total calories and thereby losing weight, by exercise that results in weight loss, by reducing intake of saturated fats and cholesterol, and perhaps by exercise alone, even without weight loss. For most people, weight loss is the first and most important action. If, after all this, the cholesterol is still too high, your physician might wish to place you on cholesterol-lowering drugs, but the use of drugs is a last resort.

Clearly, weight loss is often key. That means cutting dietary fat and calories. At the same time, increased consumption of unsaturated fats by using more corn oil, sunflower-seed oil, or safflower-seed oil in margarine and salad dressings seems prudent and may be as important as the actual loss of weight. In cooking, we recommend Pam Cooking Spray. You don't need much of this spray-on vegetable oil; it tastes just fine, and it has no sodium or cholesterol.

For weight loss, there are probably two major techniques. One is learning the caloric content of foods, the other is willpower. That means learning to say no. Just think of the number of times we eat food on airlines, even though we are not hungry, just because the food is included in the price of the ticket. Saying no is indeed difficult, and the first no is most difficult. After the first exercise of willpower, it becomes progressively easier.

For those with high cholesterol levels and/or low HDL levels who just do not wish to attempt weight loss, a dietary reduction in saturated fat and cholesterol with a commensurate increase in polyunsaturated fats might, if followed rigorously, reduce the cholesterol to a satisfactory level. Foods particularly high in polyunsaturated or monounsaturated fats are included in table 5.

There is now a lot of confusion about polyunsaturated and monounsaturated fats. A low-fat diet is ordinarily high in polyunsaturated fats, as the amount of fish, soft margarines, and salads is increased. If the polyunsaturated fats in the diet are increased markedly, cholesterol levels decline, but so may the blood levels of high-density lipoproteins (HDL). These effects could be counterbalancing. The solution of many nutritionists is to reduce the saturated fats, but keep a 1:1 ratio between monounsaturated fats (such as olive oil) and polyunsaturated fats.

So, at present, in a weight-control diet, unsaturated fats should be increased, but the optimum ratio between polyunsaturated and monounsaturated fats in that diet remains uncertain. Still, there is nothing wrong with using an olive oil dressing at least some of the time on your daily salad (as well as on the potato you are about to bake, or in marinades). You are going to use some dressing anyway, and if it turns out that olive oil is not as beneficial as some researchers think, you will have lost nothing.

Interest in fish oils as a preventive for coronary heart disease is sweeping the United States. It is the omega-3 and omega-6 fatty acids (eicosapentenoic and linoleic acids) that are thought to be the beneficial substances, acting by their anticlotting activities. An often-quoted study on this subject is by Daan Kromhout, Ph.D., and colleagues, published in the *New England Journal of Medicine* for May 9, 1985. Eight hundred and fifty-two middle-aged men were followed, starting in 1960. During the next twenty years, seventy-eight died of coronary heart disease. Fish intake was measured once in 1960. Those eating an average of thirty grams of fish a day had less than half the risk of dying of coronary heart disease.

TABLE 5

Foods That Contain Fats That Are Primarily . . .

Polyunsaturated	Monosaturated and Saturated Equally	
White fish	Lean beef	
Soft margarine	Pork	
Corn oil	Veal	
Cottonseed oil		
Soybean oil		
Safflower oil*		
Walnuts		

Monounsaturated	Saturated	
Olive oil	Whole milk	Ice cream
Peanut butter	Cream	Salami
Peanut oil	Cheese	Coconut oil
Avocado	Butter	Potato chips
Safflower oil*	Eggs	Regular
	Duck	yogurt†

NOTE: Only foods containing a substantial amount of fat have been included; low-fat foods such as chicken, turkey, etc., are therefore not considered.

*Different safflower oils can be either predominantly polyunsaturated or primarily monounsaturated.

†Skimmed-milk yogurt has saturated fats removed.

The authors noted that "the consumption of as little as one or two fish dishes per week may be of preventive value in relation to coronary heart disease."

The health food stores, among others, have gone wild selling fish oil capsules. Before going overboard, the following should be noted:

- The number of deaths analyzed was small.
- Benefit was noted in those taking one to fourteen grams a day. That is less than a quarter of a pound a week. That is very little fish.
- Even the thirty-grams-a-day amount is less than a half pound a week.
- One other study is supportive, but three reasonably good studies are negative, showing no such benefit of fish. For example, one solid study from Norway, published in 1987, compared a coastal population with inland dwellers; the coastal dwellers ate three times as much fish (about two pounds a week), but the coronary heart disease mortality over a ten-year period was actually greater than found among those who lived inland and ate much less fish.

Eating oily fish is probably a good idea as part of a balanced diet, but whether eating fish one or two times a week really reduces heart disease mortality will have to await further studies. This also applies to the omega fish oils; whether they will be useful, how much must be ingested to be effective, what adverse effects will be found—all these questions should be answered in the next five years. At present, no specific recommendation can be made.

The fish oils, the omega-3 and omega-6 polyunsaturated fatty acids, may be popular among the diet faddists and entrepreneurs, but there is a lot of evidence to enable us to state dogmatically that there is no proof they work. In addition, there is some real concern about potential adverse effects. The dosage of oils in the fish oil capsules used to attempt to lower cholesterol levels is quite large; other blood fats may be adversely affected, and there is the possibility that these fish oils may increase the risk of stroke. Fish or fish oil may be beneficial, but the value of fish oils may also be greatly exaggerated. Surely fish is a sensible component of a healthy diet, but that is about as far as we can go at present.

Although the role of fish oils in preventing heart disease is uncertain, there is a very exciting recent study. The coronary blood vessels of the heart may get narrowed by arteriosclerosis (stenosis). They can be opened up by threading a catheter with a balloon into the closed blood vessels and then repeatedly inflating the balloon (coronary angioplasty). A major problem is that in up to 40 percent of cases, the blood vessel rapidly again becomes markedly narrowed. The success or failure of the procedure can be evaluated by injecting a dye into the blood vessels and then taking pictures of the treated coronary vessels (angiography). In the September 22, 1988, issue of the *New England Journal of Medicine,* Gregory J. Dehmer, M.D., and his colleagues at the Dallas Veterans Administration Medical Center reported that administration of omega-3 (fish-oil-derived) fatty acids reduced the likelihood of restenosis by an impressive 77 percent during a three- to four-month follow-up period after the angioplasty.

This is an interesting study, but nobody should overinterpret the result. It is preliminary and applies only to people who already have severe coronary heart disease; it has nothing to do with prevention of coronary heart disease in apparently healthy people.

If the HDL levels are low, there are three separate actions that can be taken to raise the blood level: stop smoking; lose weight; and exercise. Each action may independently raise the HDL. Of course, for those who are already underweight (or in the lower part of the normal range) and do not smoke, there is only exercise, which may or may not help. Taking a couple of alcoholic drinks may raise the HDL somewhat, but that is hardly a recommendation that can be made as public health policy since one of three persons taking alcohol daily will at some time develop alcohol-related problems. Besides, it is not clear that the type of HDL elevated by alcohol is the protective type, and it has not been shown that alcohol-induced changes actually reduce heart attack risk. Nevertheless, alcohol does appear to raise the HDL to a modest degree.

An interesting study from Finland about a new HDL-raising drug appeared in the *Journal of the American Medical Association* of August 5, 1988. The drug, gemfibrozil, also lowered cholesterol levels and reduced heart attack frequency. Confirmatory studies are needed, but it seems likely that gemfibrozil or something similar will give us a much needed drug that will predictably raise HDL levels. If women still have low HDL levels after weight loss, exercise, and smoking cessation, estrogen therapy may result in substantial elevation in HDL level.

Estrogen raises a fraction of HDL called HDL_2, the part of HDL thought to be of prime importance in preventing heart attacks and coronary heart disease. Do we have enough data to actually recommend estrogen therapy? The answer is clearly no. We do not know how predictably effective estrogens might be and whether any estrogen-induced increase in HDL actually will prevent coronary heart disease and heart attacks.

A somewhat different approach is to focus more on the cholesterol:HDL ratio. If the HDL is low and the level does not increase, it can be counterbalanced by a lowering of the cholesterol which in turn will lower the cholesterol:HDL ratio. If the ratio is lowered to less than $4^1/2$ or 5, that may be as important as increasing the HDL. Weight loss and exercise should reduce the cholesterol level in most instances, even if no increase in HDL occurs. If the ratio is still unsatisfactory, a low-cholesterol, low-fat diet may reduce the cholesterol further, thus lowering the cholesterol:HDL ratio.

The approach to high blood pressure depends on the height of the blood pressure and the age of the person. The approach to a modestly elevated blood pressure in a person with no complaints related to that blood pressure is weight loss, and if that doesn't work, the next step is a weight-reduction diet together with exercise to help in the weight loss. For most people, the recommended dietary restrictions are not particularly harsh: cut down on snacks; reduce portion size at regular meals; reduce intake of rich foods, gravies, ice cream, cakes, butter; limit or eliminate alcohol consumption; and so forth.

TABLE 6

Weight Control and Low-Fat, Low-Cholesterol Foods

To Be Mostly Avoided	To Be Used in Moderation	Always Permissible
Deep-fried chicken	Lean beef	Chicken
Frankfurter	Veal	Turkey
Sausage	Lobster	White fish
Hamburger	Shrimp	Tuna fish
Salami	Crab	Cottage cheese
Calf's liver	Lamb	(skimmed-milk
Pork	Most cheeses	type)
Duck	Mashed potatoes	Most cereals
Sweetbreads	Beer and wine	Macaroni
Ham	Peanuts	Spaghetti
Regular beef	Herring	Bread
Bacon		Vegetables
Eggs		Fruits
Whole milk		Margarine
Cream		Salads
Butter		French-fried
Avocados		potatoes (if
Cakes		fried in corn or
Pies		peanut oil)
Pork chops		
Chocolate		
Ice cream		

The general outlines of a weight-control diet are summarized in table 6. I believe in gradual weight loss—one to two pounds a week—until the goal is reached. Very rapid weight loss is rarely needed, is usually not sustained, and can sometimes be dangerous.

If weight loss is not successful, the next step is to reduce salt intake.

Although there is a general agreement that salt plays some role in hypertension, exactly what it does and how has not been precisely defined. In primitive societies that consume very little salt, high blood pressure is a rarity. There are, of course, so many differences between primitive and more sophisticated societies that the lack of high blood pressure in the more primitive societies does not mean that salt is unequivocally the culprit. In the United States, a great many people whose daily intake of salt is gargantuan do not become hypertensive, and often reduction in salt intake will not control high blood pressure. Nevertheless, salt intake is felt to be important and reduction in salt consumption might be useful for the patient with hypertension.

We used to think that the sodium in salt was the culprit (salt is sodium chloride), but Dr. Norman M. Kaplan, writing in the *Annals of Internal Medicine* in March 1985 on the nondrug treatment of hypertension, pointed out that some studies now suggest the chloride may be equally or even more important.

There are three ways of reducing salt intake. One is to stop adding table salt to food. There are lots of ways to season food without adding salt, and after a while the preference for salt usually disappears. The second attack on unneeded salt is to avoid foods that contain an inordinate amount of salt. The good and bad foods in this regard are listed in table 7. The third is to avoid over-the-counter medications that have considerable amounts of salt. These are listed in table 8.

If all this does not effect reduction in blood pressure, then referral for possible attempts at stress reduction might be tried. Dr. Kaplan's review noted that the results were conflicting—six studies showed that relaxation and stress reduction decreased blood pressure, whereas three found no such effect. Clearly, it is not possible at present to make a judgment.

If the systolic blood pressure on repeated measurements is over 164 in a person under age fifty or over 179 in a person

TABLE 7

Low-Salt (Sodium) Diet

Acceptable Foods	Foods to Be Largely Avoided or Limited
Most vegetables (except broccoli, cabbage, cauliflower)	Bacon, ham
Fruits	Sausages, tongue, frankfurters
Macaroni (home-prepared with low-sodium items)	Salami
Spaghetti (home-prepared)	Most cheeses
Low-salt breads	Salted butter, margarine
Low-salt cheeses	Breads and rolls
Sweet butter, salt-free margarine	Pickles
Rice	Tomato juice
Meats (if not salted in processing, e.g., canned beef, etc.)	Anchovy paste
Most fish	Most biscuits
Chicken	Olives
Turkey	Pizza
Potatoes	Canned soups and foods
Beans, legumes (home-prepared)	Sauerkraut
Canned vegetables without salt	Shrimp, lobster, herring, crab
Home-baked yeast products	Salt pork
	Corned beef
	Ham hocks, fatback
	Salted or smoked fish
	Canned vegetables
	Most seasonings (e.g., sauces)
	Soy sauce
	MSG (Accent)
	Garlic and onion salt
	Catsup, mustard
	Potato chips

TABLE 8

Sodium Content (Approximate) of Some Nonprescription Drugs

Drug	Milligrams Sodium
Bisodol powder, 1 packet	1,500
Alka-Seltzer, 2 tablets	1,000
Sal hepatica, 1 dose	1,000
Bromo Seltzer, 1.25 gram	700
Metamucil, 1 packet	250
Rolaids, 2 tablets	100
Aspirin, 2 tablets	50
Tums, 2 tablets	40
Milk of magnesia, 1 tablespoon	35
Maalox or Gelusil, 1/2 tablespoon	20
Mylanta II, liquid, 2 tablespoons	20

over age fifty, or if the diastolic pressure is over 94, then the individual must be carefully supervised by a physician. Even here, if the diastolic pressure is less than 105 or the systolic less than 200, the physician may wish to try weight reduction and decreased salt intake before turning to blood-pressure-lowering drugs.

Stroke

The incidence of stroke in the United States has fallen more than 50 percent in the last few decades. The risk factor that dwarfs all the others is high blood pressure. One of the best studies regarding stroke and coronary heart disease is the renowned Framingham study. This seminal investigation was initiated in 1950 and involved 5,209 men and women, ages thirty to fifty-nine, who were followed for a minimum of twenty years to assess the occurrence of coronary heart disease and stroke. They found that only 15 percent of persons suffering from stroke had entirely normal blood pressure. The other 85 percent had at least some elevation of either the systolic or diastolic components.

For many years, the medical profession thought that hypertension, as it related to stroke, could be divided into two categories: mild to moderate hypertension, defined as a diastolic pressure of 90 mm Hg to 104 mm Hg; and severe hypertension, defined as a diastolic pressure of 105 mm Hg or greater. There was very good evidence provided by studies carried out under the purview of the Veterans Administration that reducing the blood pressure in persons with severe hypertension reduced the likelihood of subsequent stroke. But there was no convincing study to show that control of mild hypertension reduced the frequency of stroke. Now there is persuasive evidence from several studies that treatment of mild to moderate high blood pressure is also beneficial. For example, a study conducted in fourteen centers around the United States over a five-year period of persons with mild to moderate high blood pressure has shown a very substantial reduction in stroke occurrence among those whose blood pressure was well controlled compared with those who were less vigorously treated and whose blood pressure was less well controlled. It is interesting that treatment of mild to moderate hypertension clearly reduces the incidence of stroke, but the evidence that such treatment reduces the incidence of heart attacks is less impressive.

What about other risk factors for stroke? Cholesterol levels are related to stroke in some age categories, but the relationship is not very impressive. Diabetes is a risk factor, but there is currently no evidence that control of the diabetes changes the likelihood of stroke. In other words, if you have diabetes, you are more likely to get a stroke, but controlling the diabetes by diet and taking insulin probably won't change that likelihood.

Most studies have not shown a clear relationship between smoking and stroke occurrence and the studies on smoking and brain blood flow suggest that only heavy smoking will be related to stroke occurrence. The difficulty in making a firm statement is illustrated by contrasting views in two good studies. One by Lennart Welin, M.D., and his colleagues from Gothenburg and Uppsala universities in Sweden investigated risk factors for stroke in a group of men born in 1913. Smoking in any amount did not increase the risk of stroke. On the other hand, Philip A. Wolf and his colleagues, writing in the *Journal of the American Medical Association,* in February 1988, about the men and women enrolled in the Framingham heart study, reported that smoking increased the risk of stroke in both men and women to a moderate extent. There was clear evidence of a dose-response relationship; smoking a half pack or less a day hardly increased the risk at all, but smoking two packs a day doubled the risk of stroke. Among those who stopped smoking, the increased risk disappeared within two to five years. This is probably the best of the studies. Smoking is not nearly so important a risk factor for stroke as high blood pressure, but it does seem to be a risk factor. At present, the data suggest that smoking more than one pack a day is bad for brain function in some persons and may result in increased strokes. That is as far as one can go with the available information.

The *New England Journal of Medicine* in January 1987 suggested that higher potassium intake protected against stroke. That interesting but very preliminary study will probably get a lot of people to increase their intake of potassium-containing foods or even take potassium supplements. But that would be premature. Very small numbers of stroke cases were involved, and the results were statistically significant only for women. The role of less potassium intake in promoting stroke or the role of increased potassium intake in preventing stroke is at present just not known.

According to Swedish investigators, there are two other possibly important risk factors for stroke. One is abdominal obesity (an increased ratio of abdominal girth to hip circumference) and the other is the amount of clotting factor fibrinogen in the blood. We need more information about these measurements as neither is adequately documented.

Cancer Prevention

Some components of the Health-Full-Life Program are related to cancer prevention. Most fit into the category of secondary prevention, or early intervention.

Smoking Do not smoke or, if you must smoke, limit that smoking to less than ten cigarettes a day.

Tobacco smoking is the main risk factor for lung cancer. What is not appreciated enough is that this is very much dose-related. For a man, the lifetime risk of lung cancer is 1 in 11, but the risk is minuscule if you do not smoke and it is much higher if you smoke two to four packs a day. The obvious question is what amount of smoking, if any, is safe. There is no evidence that one to two cigarettes per day can cause lung cancer. The likelihood of cancer does increase as the smoker moves up to a pack a day, but the increased risk at a half pack a day or less is very small.

Of the approximately 100,000 cases of cancer of the lung each year that can be attributed mainly to cigarette smoking, only 3,000 to 5,000 cases will occur in those smoking less than a half pack a day. Unfortunately, only 25 percent of smokers limit themselves to less than a half pack a day.

If you do choose to smoke and wish to reduce the risk of developing cancer, should you purchase only low-tar brands? The answer is unequivocally yes. Cigarettes are modified by changing the tobacco content of tars and other substances or by adding filters. The evidence that low-tar cigarettes reduce the likelihood of cancer is considerable. Several studies in the United States, England, and Finland show that use of filtered low-tar cigarettes reduces the risk of lung cancer by one-third to one-half. If you have to smoke and you know smoking is potentially harmful, surely it makes sense to reduce the health risks as much as possible. Confine the amount to less than a half pack per day, use filters, and smoke only low-tar cigarettes. Surprisingly, as of 1986, only about half of the cigarettes consumed in the U.S. were the low-tar variety. I personally feel that high-tar, high-nicotine cigarettes ought to be banned.

I should stress that there are two components to smoking-related lung cancer risk: the number of cigarettes you smoke each day and how many years you have smoked. Of the two, duration is more important. If you smoke a given number of cigarettes for ten years, the risk is much greater than smoking the same amount for five years. Although duration of smoking is more critical than dose, it is important to realize that doubling the number of cigarettes used per day from, say, ten to twenty or twenty to forty will double the risk of lung cancer.

What about the reduction in risk of lung cancer after stopping smoking? Some say the risk gradually decreases, so ten years after stopping cigarettes your risk is no greater than the nonsmoker. Richard Peto, a talented British epidemiologist, is less optimistic. He feels that stopping avoids the further and escalating risk from continued smoking, but that the risk will still be greater than for those who never smoked.

Air pollution frequently is condemned as contributing to lung cancer, and there are some studies supporting that hypothesis. For example, when the enormous amount of industrially caused pollution in London was markedly reduced, lung cancer rates fell about 20 percent, even though there was no evidence of a change in smoking patterns. At present, there is no firm evidence that most air pollutants can, in themselves, induce lung cancer in the absence of smoking. However, certain air pollutants can increase the cancer-producing potential of tobacco.

One air pollutant that has caused a great deal of recent concern in regard to lung cancer is radon, a very dangerous carcinogenic substance that is, for the most part, not caused by man. Rather, it is found in certain geographic areas and gets into houses whose foundations are dug into those soils. It could well turn out to be a significant factor for lung cancer among those who do not smoke and it, like asbestos, may markedly increase the likelihood of lung cancer in smokers—that is, radon and tobacco together, like asbestos and tobacco, may act synergistically and profoundly increase the risk to smokers. Indeed, one very good argument against smoking even one half pack a day or less is that smoking fewer than ten cigarettes a day may not by itself be enough to induce lung cancer, but combined with exposure to asbestos or radon, even that limited amount of smoking may be dangerous.

Can passive smoking cause lung cancer in nearby nonsmokers? A modest number of studies purport to show that passive smoking can cause lung cancer. Among the most quoted studies, one from Japan and one from Greece have obvious major flaws. One critic pointed out that in the Japanese study, the amount inhaled passively by wives of smokers would be equivalent to one cigarette per day, an amount that would almost certainly not cause lung cancer. A third study, published September 10, 1983, in the British journal *Lancet,* is better but still creates difficulties in interpretation. No relationship was found for passive smoking if the spouse smoked less than two packs per day. A study by the American Cancer Society group headed by Lawrence Garfinkel, published in the *Journal of the National Cancer Institute* in September 1985, found that if the husband of a nonsmoking wife smoked at least two packs a day, there was a moderately increased risk of lung cancer for the wife that was statistically significant. So if there is any potential for passive smoking to cause cancer, it is only if the person has close contact with a very heavy smoker for a long time.

Other observers insist that nonsmokers exposed constantly to heavy smokers absorb the equivalent of one to nine cigarettes a day and therefore are at the same risk as light smokers. According to an article by a Swedish group published in the *American Journal of Epidemiology* in January 1987, that increased risk is between 100 and 900 percent. But those figures need some explication. The risk for a nonsmoking woman is tiny; so an increase of severalfold in risk is still very, very small. As noted in the *American Journal of Epidemiology* article: "It is obvious that lung cancer in passive smokers is a rare phenomenon."

As far as I am concerned, the role of passive smoking remains uncertain and, as I have indicated, not proven at all for exposure to the smoke of an individual smoking less than a half pack a day. If there is a problem, it is either exposure to a single heavy smoker or simultaneously to two or more heavy smokers either in the house or in a closed environment at the workplace.

Since passive smoking is, at most, equivalent to smoking less than a half pack a day, the problem of passive smoking and possible cancer could probably be solved entirely by a law that would prohibit the manufacture or sale of any cigarette other than those that are low-tar and filtered. That would protect the public from potential lung cancer from passive smoking and still allow those who insist on smoking to do so.

So the evidence on passive smoking, taking all the studies together, is not very impressive. Is there still reason for concern? I think the answer is probably yes. As I indicated in the section on heart disease, my concern is the additive effects of multiple toxins, each in small concentration. Most of us are exposed to multiple toxins, some naturally occurring, some man-made. The list of substances we may be exposed to is endless—radon from rock formations, asbestos from construction sites, the effluent of garbage incinerators and factories, the exhaust of cars, radioactivity from nuclear plants or nuclear accidents. Some airborne toxins can be carried for hundreds or thousands of miles. A single individual might inhale a welter of toxic substances in any given day, each of which, considered alone, would be in concentration that was considered to be in the safe range, but acting together may cause mischief.

To prove these pollutants acting together can cause lung cancer is very difficult. At present, there is no such proof, and there may not be for decades. And that means we must act prudently, using common sense. Common sense would dictate that we keep the air we breathe as free of toxic substances as possible. We should eliminate as much radon from our homes as we can, control car exhausts, minimize incinerator and smokestack effluents and minimize the amount of smoke we inhale from cigarettes.

I don't smoke. I am not afraid that the smoke I inhale from the cigarettes of others will give me cancer. But I am concerned that all the junk we so casually spew into the air, of which cigarette smoke is a part, taken together and acting in concert may be hazardous to my health—and to yours.

Thus far, the campaign by the various antismoking groups has met with substantial success. In 1963, prior to the surgeon general's report warning of the health hazards of smoking, cigarette consumption was 516 billion cigarettes, or over 4,300 cigarettes for each adult over eighteen years of age. That amounts to 215 packs of cigarettes for every adult in a single year. Since the surgeon general's report, the most impressive reduction has been among adult males. In 1955 and 1956, more than 50 percent of men smoked; by 1975, this percentage had fallen to 39; and by 1985, the percentage of adult male smokers had fallen to 33 percent. The trend among women is less encouraging. In 1955, 24 percent smoked. By 1965, this had increased to 34.4 percent; but 20 years later, in 1985, the percentage of smokers had fallen to 28 percent. In 1983, cigarette consumption fell to 600 billion cigarettes, a 40 billion decrease from the 1981 peak. That's still about 180 packs per year per capita, but it is now estimated that only 32 percent of male adults and 28 percent of female adults smoke and there are estimated 33 million adult ex-smokers. Even more encouraging are data showing that the rate of increased deaths from smoking-related lung cancer has slowed markedly in men; among men under forty-five years of age, the rate has actually fallen.

Pap Smears The Pap smear is both primary and secondary prevention, and should be done every two years after age twenty. Cervical cancer usually develops quite slowly, in three stages. First, the cells of the cervix, the lowest part of the womb, become abnormal. This change is called dysplasia; in most cases, dysplasia never progresses to cancer, but it is still a risk factor for cancer; finding it by Pap smear and removing those dysplastic cells is primary prevention. The second step in the progression is totally localized, noninvasive cancer, called "cancer in situ." If discovered by a Pap smear in that stage, the earliest cancer stage, it can easily be removed; that is secondary prevention. Cancer in situ of the cervix may occasionally regress spontaneously, may remain in situ without ever progressing to invasive cancer, or may develop into invasive cancer; change into invasive cancer can occur very quickly or may take many years.

The evidence available today indicates that cervical cancer is caused by a virus. A decade ago, the virus implicated was a member of the herpes group, but now most attention is focused on papilloma viruses. Although cause-and-effect has not been proved fully, it would seem very likely that these viruses will turn out to be the major cause of cervical cancer.

If a given Pap smear is negative, there is no reason to get another for two years. (If the Pap smear shows any abnormalities, it should be done yearly and, of course, if it shows a local tumor growth, the tumor should be taken care of immediately.) Even if a local tumor starts within two years, it will almost invariably stay localized for a considerable time. Thus, a two-year interval is perfectly reasonable. Cancer of the cervix almost never occurs in sexually inactive women, so if every woman in the United States who is or has been sexually active had a Pap smear done every two years, we would virtually wipe out invasive cancer of the cervix. It is inexcusable for thousands of women to continue to die of this disease every year.

I would stress that the Pap smear, developed by Dr. George Papanicolaou, is simple, painless, and effective. The cervix, the lowest portion of the uterus, is only a few inches from the entrance to the vagina. A smear is taken from the cervix and the cells in the smear are examined under the microscope; normal cells, inflammatory cells, early cancer, and invasive cancer can be detected. There are now multiple studies documenting the efficacy of the Pap smear.

Among the many supportive studies is one published September 21, 1984, in the *Journal of the American Medical Association.* Swedish investigators followed 200,000 women for 10 years and found a 75 percent drop in the incidence of invasive cervical cancer if a woman had a Pap smear at least once in that ten-year period. They estimated that if every woman had a Pap smear every three years, about 90 percent of invasive cervical cancer would be avoided. My own feeling is that with the Health-Full-Life schedule of a Pap smear every two years, well over 90 percent could be avoided.

The argument for stopping Pap screening at age sixty or sixty-five appears to me to be very weak. About one-third of all cases of cervical cancer are detected after age sixty, and one out of every four is diagnosed after age sixty-five. To me, the prudent recommendation is a Pap test every other year until at least age seventy-five.

Breast Self-examination Starting at age thirty, every woman should examine her own breasts monthly and have them examined yearly by an expert.

About 70 to 80 percent of lumps in the breast are discovered by women themselves—and early discovery is the key to a high cure rate. Some women do not examine their breasts because they are afraid of what they will find. But there is less reason for fear than one might think—if a lump *is* found, the chances are very good that it is benign, not malignant.

Self-examination is quick and easy. In a sitting position in front of a mirror, the woman should examine her breasts visually with her shoulders back, looking for irregularities, skin dimpling or puckering, or changes in the nipple, in particular, retraction. Then, in a sitting and later in a recumbent position, she should carefully palpate each quadrant of each breast, moving her hands slowly from area to area and feeling first superficially and then deeply; the latter should create a feeling of pressure and even slight discomfort. If the woman feels any lump or irregularity, she should consult a physician. It is also a good idea at the beginning for a woman to examine her own breasts under supervision of a nurse practitioner or physician.

Self-examination should be done between menstrual periods. The breasts become engorged just prior to and during the menstrual period and this normal engorgement can mistakenly be interpreted as a tumor.

It is important to do breast self-examination not only to find an early cancer, but also to detect noncancerous lumps so that these can be followed closely, since such benign growths can lead to cancer. If such growths are adequately followed, they can, if necessary, be removed before cancer develops or as soon as a cancerous change takes place, before spread can occur. The point is that the benign, noncancerous lumps alert the woman and the physician to be on the lookout for cancer. She has a greater risk of cancer, but once the lumps are detected and observed carefully, she also has a very great chance of detecting any cancer very early when it is localized and curable.

Again, I would emphasize that most lumps are not cancer; they merely warn that the woman must have regular surveillance to make sure that cancer does not develop, or if it should occur, that it can be treated promptly before it spreads.

The early detection of breast cancer is, of course, secondary prevention. We do not know the cause of breast cancer or how to prevent it.

It is of interest that a Gallup poll published in 1984 showed that half of adult women examine their breasts for lumps at least three times a year, but only a quarter do it monthly, and many of these probably carry out the examination improperly. No wonder studies of self-examination are not encouraging.

I know a woman who is small-breasted and says she did regular self-examinations. One day, she saw striking breast distortion and ten days later a large tumor was removed. It had obviously been there for months (or even years) and should have been easy to palpate. Why did she miss it on self-examination? Almost surely she, like perhaps half the people doing self-examination, was subconsciously afraid of finding the tumor, and even though she had been carefully instructed in the technique of self-examination, she performed the test in a slipshod fashion, subconsciously trying not to find an abnormal lump. We have to persuade women that treatment is now effective enough that careful self-examination makes sense and that early detection really does save lives and misery. An interesting preliminary study by a group from the University of Washington in Seattle presented at the Society for Epidemiologic Research meeting in June 1987 suggested real benefit in avoiding serious breast cancer for women who performed thorough self-examination compared with those who did inadequate or superficial examinations.

There are still those who question whether breast examination should be recommended as public health policy. It seems to me that the evidence favors such examinations, but critics mention five serious reasons for being skeptical. First, self-examination is not sensitive enough; it misses too many tumors. That is true, but, in part, this can be attributed to women not doing self-examination correctly. Second, it is not specific; most lumps found are not cancer. Although again this is true, it is also important to find noncancerous lumps that might become cancerous. Third, the mammogram is a better test. It is, but it misses up to 20 percent of tumors; in some cases, self-examination shows a tumor when the mammogram missed it. Fourth, if a lump is found, it represents a tumor that has been there a long time and is well advanced. I do not accept this point. The evidence that the tumor must have been there a long time is based on animal studies of growth of breast cancer cells. Those studies may not be relevant to human breast cancer. In any case, the evidence shows that the smaller the tumor when it is detected, the better the long-term survival rate. The final point relates to the absence of a controlled trial, that is, following a large group of women for the occurrence of breast cancer over a period of many years, half of whom did self-examination and half of whom did not. That would be impossible (and unethical) to do now.

The debate about the usefulness of self-examination of the breast (SBE) will rage for a long time. The most pessimistic view is that by the time a woman feels a lump, the malignancy will already have spread to other tissues, although the evidence of such spread may not appear for many years. The opposing, optimistic view is that early detection by a woman can prevent dissemination of the cancer. In the April 24, 1987, issue of the *Journal of the American Medical Association,* Michael O'Malley and Suzanne Fletcher, M.D., writing for the U.S. Preventive Services Task Force, a highly reputable and careful group, challenged the usefulness of SBE.

There is one reasonable study showing that among a cohort of women, those who did SBE had fewer deaths from breast cancer and increased five-year survival rates, but O'Malley and Fletcher noted that there were very few adequate studies. They pointed out that the available information indicates that SBE has a sensitivity of only 20 to 30 percent—if a woman has a breast cancer, the likelihood of finding it by SBE is only 2 or 3 out of 10. That is not very good. And, too often, lumps that are detected by SBE and are thought to be cancer turn out to be noncancerous. Proving they are noncancerous can be quite costly.

O'Malley and Fletcher concluded: "Breast self-examination has potential as a screening test for breast cancer, but many questions require scientific examination before this procedure can be advocated as a screening test for breast cancer."

As soon as the report was published, a lot of experts, including representatives of the American Cancer Society and the National Cancer Institute, sprang to the defense of SBE. The general feeling seems to be that we should not abandon SBE, but we wish it were a more effective technique.

Interestingly, and to me surprisingly, O'Malley and Fletcher gave some reasonably strong endorsement to annual physical examination by a physician or trained nurse. I, personally, do not feel the evidence is either better or worse for the yearly examination than for SBE.

All in all, I think the evidence supports breast self-examination. In future years, we may well develop a technique that is reasonable in cost and that will make self-examination obsolete. But right now, self-examination, yearly examination by an expert, and mammography are the best we have available. Women should take advantage of all of these.

There is another important point emphasized to me by Dr. Frank Gump, a renowned breast cancer expert at Columbia Presbyterian Hospital in New York City. He is a surgeon and notes that the smaller the size of the lump, the more likely it is that a limited operation, a lumpectomy, can be performed, removing the lump and surrounding tissues, but preserving the breast. That alone makes it worthwhile for women to learn to perform SBE correctly so that tumors can be detected as early as possible.

Mammography Every woman over age forty should not only examine her breasts, but should also have a mammographic examination at least every other year and preferably yearly.

When a mammogram is done, the radiologist is looking for tiny calcifications and for an irregular lump. A modification of mammography is xerography. It is very similar, gives a more dramatic picture, but entails a bit more radiation. No other procedure can detect a breast cancer at such an early stage. If the tumor is found by a mammogram but cannot be felt, and then is removed, the cure rate appears to be over 90 percent. That is much better than the cure rate if a cancer is found by feeling a lump and then removing the cancer. So it is best to detect the cancer at its earliest stages by mammography, next best to find it when it is small by feeling the lump, and worst not to detect the lump until it is quite large.

There are some important questions regarding mammography:

- *Is it virtually infallible?* The answer is no. About 10 to 20 percent of breast cancers are missed by mammography. Some are felt and the mammogram still does not pick them up. Others appear in the one-year interval between mammograms; many of these have been missed on the first mammogram since most breast tumors do grow slowly, but in some cases, the evidence suggests the tumor was a very rapid-growing cancer. The problem in that situation would be with the rapidity of growth of the cancer, not with the mammogram.

- *If a growth is found, is it always cancer?* Assuming the mammogram is interpreted competently, 70 to 80 percent of masses that look like cancer are cancer, but 20 to 30 percent are not. If all lumps found on mammography (those that look like cancer, those that are somewhat suspicious, and those that look benign) are added together, then only about 20 percent of all growths found by mammography plus breast examination turn out to be cancer.

- *Can a yearly mammogram itself cause breast cancer?* The amount of radiation to each breast is now well under 0.2 rad, an amount so small that the chances of its causing cancer are tiny. There is at present *no* evidence that a yearly mammogram can cause cancer. Conceivably, it could. If the worst-case estimates are used, the number of cancers per 1 million women studied each year for forty years would be 180 to 1,200 cancers. That unproved, worst-case extrapolation is balanced against the grim fact that 1 in 10 women will get breast cancer in a lifetime and the only hope of early enough detection to get a very high cure rate is the mammogram. So the risk of radiation-induced cancer from mammography is tiny (and may not exist at all) and the potential benefits are enormous.

- *Is the evidence clear that mammography should be done in women forty years of age and older rather than wait until age fifty?* There are some good studies showing definite benefit in saving lives in the forty–to–forty-nine–year age group. There are also some studies that show no benefit in that age group. The Canadian Task Force on the Periodic Health Examination is perhaps the most respected group in the world in regard to evaluation of screening activities. In the April 1, 1986, issue of the *Canadian Medical Association Journal,* they indicated they still felt unsure about the efficacy of mammography in the forty–to–forty-nine age group. The study most quoted is one formulated by Health Insurance Plan (HIP) in New York City. Using a crude mammography machine more than twenty years ago in a large study involving more than twenty thousand women, the HIP group found definite benefit for those over fifty years of age; but the results for those aged forty to forty-nine were unclear. Now there has been time for an eighteen-to-twenty-year follow-up. The encouraging results were presented in June 1988 at the annual meeting of the Society for Epidemiologic Research; with prolonged follow-up, reduced deaths from breast cancer were found in all women over age forty.

The biggest problem with mammography is the cost. In some areas, each test can cost $120 to $200. That is outrageously high. In the Health-Full-Life Program, we have budgeted $60 to $80 for a mammograph; as of 1989, that is reasonable and we expect no difficulty in getting good radiologists to do the study for that amount or less.

The mammogram is questionably cost-effective. If you balance the cost of breast cancer versus the cost of the mammogram program, the costs, according to a study done for Health-Full-Life, are about equal. The costs of the breast cancer include treatment, lost productivity, costs to a company to train a new worker, etc. The costs of the mammogram program are considerable because a given company, or health insurance carrier, or group of individuals must pay for all the negative tests as well as the expenses for taking out growths that turn out not to be cancer. It then comes down to whether we wish to pay for saving lives; mammograms will save lives, but the screening program is not inexpensive.

Many experts feel that a woman with a family history (mother, sister) of breast cancer should have a screening mammogram between the ages of thirty-five and forty. Others think that all women should have one screening mammogram between ages thirty-five and forty. The recommendation makes sense for a woman with a family history of breast cancer in close relatives even though the efficacy of such a test is ill-documented and breast cancer is still infrequent before age forty. For women with no such family history, the screening mammogram between ages thirty-five and forty is optional; it is reasonable, but the benefits are not established.

The medical profession should give specific recommendations based on our best assessment of the available data. That is why it is a bit distressing to see a recommendation in an otherwise excellent March 11, 1988, *Journal of the American Medical Association* article by acknowledged experts that says the family doctor or the woman with her family doctor should make the decision about mammography between ages forty and forty-nine. To me, that is ridiculous and a cop-out. If the authors of the study, who are experts, can't make a recommendation, how can a less well-informed family physician or the woman herself make the decision?

I will not be evasive. Herewith are my summary recommendations:

1. Every woman age thirty or older should do monthly breast self-examination. Additionally, she should learn how to find lumps using models of the breast. That may require a bit of effort. Some doctors and clinics have such models, but it may require a call to the local cancer society to find out where to go to get the proper training. Each woman should become familiar with the texture of her breasts and not be afraid of finding a lump. Finding a cancer early can only help her.
2. Each year a breast examination should be done by an expert (doctor or nurse).
3. Mammography should be done yearly, starting at age forty. A woman should shop around if the mammogram fee is more than $40 to $80.
4. A screening mammogram under age forty is optional; it is advisable if a close relative has had breast cancer.

Perhaps twenty to thirty years from now a woman will provide a blood specimen, a computerized analysis of her genes will be made, and she can be told whether she is a candidate for breast cancer. Then we can focus on a high-risk group and suggest much more limited screening for the low-risk group. By then, we may also know how to totally prevent breast cancer. And, in the interim, we will have better early detection techniques than we have now, but for the present, I believe my recommendations make good sense.

Bowel Cancer Every man and woman over age forty should have the stools (bowel movements) examined each year for blood. The logic behind this test is quite clear. The overwhelming majority of bowel tumors bleed, and this bleeding can be detected by a simple chemical test. All you have to do is collect the specimen and get it to the laboratory. As with breast cancer, it makes a great deal of difference if the tumor is found early. At the Strang Clinic in New York City, fifty-eight colon cancers were detected before there were any symptoms. The fifteen-year survival was an extraordinary 88 percent.

There are certain small growths called polyps that protrude from the wall of the bowel into the intestinal lumen. Some types of polyps can become cancerous. Since they are a risk factor for cancer, removing them is primary prevention. The blood in the stool may also indicate there is a polyp that has already changed into cancer or that there is a cancer that has developed but is unrelated to polyps. If detected early and removed, that is secondary prevention. Bowel cancer is one of the three most important cancers in frequency of occurrence and numbers of deaths in the United States; lung and breast cancer are the other two.

Unfortunately, we do not know the causes of bowel cancer other than the presence of polyps, and there is at present *no* known way of preventing bowel cancer by either avoiding some dietary constituent or adding a nutritional element or a dietary supplement.

The obvious question, then, is what is the most effective way to find tumors early, before there are symptoms such as pain and grossly evident bleeding? Once symptoms have occurred, the outlook is bleak—if gross bleeding, pain, and so forth, have been present for seven months when a bowel cancer is found, the five-year survival rate is only 25 percent; if there have been symptoms for three months, the five-year survival rate is 40 percent; but if the cancer is found by routine examination in a person without symptoms, about 90 percent survive for a prolonged time and appear cured.

There is no ideal test for detecting bowel cancer in its earliest stages. Currently, testing the stools for blood yearly is the best we have to offer. Why only after age forty? Because less than 5 percent of bowel cancers occur before that age, and in most of those, there is some known disease that has alerted the physician to the increased risk of such cancers. The best way at present to detect silent intestinal bleeding is the Hemoccult slide. This is a chemically treated slide to which a tiny amount of bowel movement is added by use of an applicator. The material on the slide is allowed to dry in air and then a drop of color developer is placed on the slide; if blood is present, within a minute a blue color is seen.

There is now great emphasis on home detection of silent bleeding by use of special toilet papers or other similar materials. No one of these has been adequately documented or tested. The percentage of false negatives due to misreading and false positives due to overreading will almost surely be quite significant. The proponents say that if there is a positive, then regular Hemoccults should be done and taken to the laboratory or physician, but in our litigious society, a wary doctor, told of a home positive, will often decide to do an expensive work-up even if the confirmatory Hemoccult is negative. In some cases, they won't even bother with a confirmatory Hemoccult. That means a big jump in costs. Home tests may indeed be useful, but they should be scrutinized very thoroughly before they are recommended.

It is critical that the test be carried out correctly. It is also important to realize that if the test is positive, it does not necessarily mean cancer. In at least 80 percent (and probably in over 90 percent) of positive tests, the patient has hemorrhoids or some other minor disease. If the test is positive, further investigation is necessary to distinguish between the nonmalignant and the malignant causes of the positive result.

One problem with the test for blood in the stools is the false negative tests that result from improper techniques. One reason for this is the failure to study three consecutive specimens. If you collect a specimen on Monday, Wednesday, and Friday, but have bowel movements each day, then the collection technique is incorrect because the bleeding can be intermittent and missed unless three specimens are submitted from consecutive bowel movements. If a person has two movements a day, then both bowel movements from one day and the first bowel movement from the next day must be examined.

The other major reason for failure to get a positive in the presence of a cancer is an incorrect diet. It is important that seventy-two hours before the day you collect specimens, you place yourself on a special diet that contains roughage that will cause the tumor to bleed. It is not a very obscure diet. It consists of white fish, ham, poultry, fruits (prunes, apples, grapes), certain vegetables (lettuce, spinach, corn), peanuts, whole grain bread and bran cereals. Red meats are not permitted because they contain blood and give false positive results.

The usual collection technique is to fish part of the bowel movement out of the toilet bowl with an applicator and place a piece of the specimen on the special slide. This collection technique is not particularly aesthetic and most people will never agree to collecting specimens in that way.

We have decided on an easier approach. Obtain the slides from your physician (or the laboratory) as well as six-inch sticks with a cotton swab at the end (obtainable at any drugstore). After a bowel movement, you apply the swab gently to the anal area before wiping with toilet paper. You do this twice with separate swabs and use separate parts of the Hemoccult slide for each swab. This is done on each of the three consecutive bowel movements. It is simple and aesthetically acceptable.

You should not take aspirin for one week prior to the Hemoccult test because aspirin can cause bleeding and give a false positive test. Vitamin C should also not be taken for a few days before the test because it can interfere with the chemicals used to carry out the test. Turnips, cantaloupe, cauliflower, horseradish, and radishes should also be avoided for seventy-two hours prior to the test because they, too, can give false positive results. Other vegetables either should be cooked or taken in moderation and other uncooked fruits should be avoided (except for oranges and strawberries).

The final point relates to speed of processing the slides. We used to think that you could collect all three, mail them to a physician, and get accurate results. This is probably not so. Within four days, a specimen that was positive when tested within forty-eight hours may become negative. Consequently, if you use Hemoccult slides, you should get them to the physician or laboratory within two days, and the slides must then be processed immediately (it takes only one minute to test each slide). Collecting three stool specimens every year starting at age forty is not much to deal with when you realize that it may mean the difference between detecting bowel cancer in an early, curable stage and waiting until the malignancy has spread and symptoms are present.

There is now a vigorous attack on tests to detect silent bleeding by the techniques I have outlined. In essence, the critics insist there are too many false positives (due to testing techniques or nontumorous lesions) and too many false negatives. They also say there has not yet been a good, properly designed clinical study. It is true that in most cases, a positive test turns out to be noncancerous, and it is also true that about 15 to 25 percent of cancers are not detected by testing for blood in the stool (these are considered false negative tests). However, if the test is done carefully, the number of false positives and false negatives can be minimized; and the older one is, the more likely it is that the cause of silent bleeding is either a polyp or a cancer. Five carefully designed studies of silent bleeding are now being carried out. When they are finished, perhaps five years from now, I may wish to modify this recommendation, but at present I am convinced that testing for silent intestinal bleeding is indicated. Preliminary results from one of these studies were published in the British journal *Lancet* (May 27, 1989). The results were very encouraging; cancers were detected in an earlier stage in those who were screened compared with controls, and by the third screening, the frequency of cancer in those tested was substantially less than was found in the controls.

Colonoscopy Men and women over age forty-five should have a left-sided colonoscopy every five years to remove polyps.

There are three types of bowel examination. The first, called rigid proctoscopy, is done with a metal tube that visualizes about ten inches. Because it is a rigid tube, it causes a lot of discomfort, and because it sees only ten inches of the intestine, it misses many polyps. It is an unpleasant procedure. I would not recommend it for this type of program—or, for that matter, for any program. Use of the rigid proctoscope is barbaric and anachronistic. Nobody should be doing it anymore. Flexible left-sided colonoscopy (sigmoidoscopy) is done with a pliable tube that reaches about twenty-five inches (sixty centimeters), visualizes many more polyps, causes very little discomfort, and is the examination I recommend. The third type of examination is called full colonoscopy. It can visualize the entire intestine (about sixty inches), but is more dangerous and more costly and thus cannot be recommended for general public health policy for persons with no symptoms; it should be used primarily as a follow-up for those found to have polyps on left-sided colonoscopy. Although I recommend the sixty-centimeter examination with a flexible instrument, it is almost as effective to do a slightly less extensive examination that visualizes thirty-five centimeters. The advantage of doing the thirty-five-centimeter examination is that it carries virtually no risk, whereas the sixty-centimeter study carries a very slight risk of perforating the intestine.

As I have indicated, a polyp is a benign tumor with a thin base that grows from the bowel wall and protrudes into the lumen of the intestine. The best evidence suggests that certain types of polyps in the large intestine may become malignant; thus, removal can prevent cancer. To remove a polyp, you place a snare over it, cut it off at the base, and stop bleeding by electrocoagulation. This is quite easy to do through the colonoscope and is not painful (though there may be some discomfort). The physician inserts the colonoscope, which has a light at the end, guides it under direct vision until he locates the polyps, and then advances a polyp-cutting snare through the colonoscope.

Dr. Victor A. Gilbertsen of the University of Minnesota Medical Center carried out multiple proctoscopies on 18,158 patients during a twenty-five-year period. At each proctoscopy, polyps were removed. In this population, seventy-five to eighty cancers would have been expected, but only eleven occurred. This was attributed to polyp removal. On the basis of this extensive and impressive experience, Gilbertsen recommended a proctoscopy every two to three years after age fifty, but writing in the journal *Cancer* in 1974, Gilbertsen himself noted, "An even longer interval may be relatively satisfactory. No patient who has discontinued annual examinations has developed a lower bowel cancer which has been diagnosed during the first seven years following examinations at the center." To me, this means that if you remove polyps every five years, that is perfectly satisfactory. This study is far from perfect, but it, along with two other imperfect studies (from Kaiser Permanente in California and the Strang Clinic in New York City), is the best we have and therefore has to be the data base for current policy.

Why a sigmoidoscopy with polyp removal only after age forty-five? Because 92 percent of all bowel cancers are detected after fifty, and many of those who get bowel cancer before age fifty have diseases that predispose them to bowel cancer and are already under special surveillance. Because polyps that become cancerous may remain silent for years, it makes sense to do left-sided colonoscopy starting at age forty-five, but start the Hemoccult tests at age forty.

Why not do a flexible colonoscopy every year to detect

more cancers early? There is no evidence that a yearly flexible colonoscopy to twenty-five inches plus Hemoccult testing for blood is any better than yearly Hemoccult tests alone, plus left-sided colonoscopy every five years, and it would be a lot more expensive: charges generally range from a minimum of $100 up to $1,000. If you don't mind the expense and the annoyance of the test, and if it makes you feel better, have a twenty-five-inch colonoscopy (or a sixty-inch colonoscopy) done every one, two, or three years. But I see no reason for doing so. A flexible colonoscopy examination every five years for polyp removal plus yearly Hemoccult studies for blood is perfectly satisfactory. Interestingly, when I proposed the every-five-years interval, I was severely criticized by those who insisted on every year. Slowly, the pendulum is shifting. First, every other year was deemed acceptable, then every three years, but I believe the evidence on slow growth of cancers and polyps will almost surely result in a five-year consensus.

The interval is important for both medical and financial reasons. If the health insurance industry and employers are expected to support prevention programs, costs and premiums must be kept reasonable, and that in turn means that expensive components of a program must be kept to the minimum needed to do the job. There is a big difference in costs between doing a colonoscopy every year or two versus every five years; and as far as I can see, there is no medical advantage to every two or three years. I find it a lot easier to adjust to the test every five years rather than every two or three years.

About 5 to 10 percent of those over age forty-five will have a polyp. If one is found, there is a 20 to 50 percent likelihood that additional polyps will be found. If a polyp is found, it is necessary to schedule the person for a full colonoscopy with polyp removal to remove any polyps beyond the range of the 60-centimeter study. A full colonoscopy is also needed if there is evidence of blood in the stool.

If a person has a polyp detected, how often should that person have colonoscopy thereafter? Some say yearly, but a preliminary study has shown no differences in detecting new polyps or cancers between groups having colonoscopies every year or every three years. Once a polyp is detected and removed, it will be necessary to have full colonoscopy every three years to find and remove any new polyps before they become cancerous. In the January 27, 1989, issue of the *Journal of the American Medical Association* there were three articles and an editorial on screening for bowel cancer; all were written by experts, but the conclusions were so divergent and unclear that they left doctors, their patients, and the general public confused. It is true that there are some important unanswered questions and there is no ideal screening program for bowel cancer, but the approach I have outlined is reasonable and not inordinately expensive. The combination of yearly Hemoccult tests for bleeding starting at age forty and flexible 60-centimeter colonoscopy every five years after age forty-five will not pick up all polyps and cancers, but it will detect the overwhelming majority. For the large majority of people who have no abnormal findings, it is very reassuring. Eventually, we will have better tests, but the Health-Full-Life approach surely makes good sense for now.

Testicular Self-examination There is one other simple self-examination that can be done by men and that is periodic examination of the testicles. Normally, there is a small mass above the testicles; this is the "epididymis" and it is perfectly normal. A lump in the testis itself is not.

Testicular tumors occur infrequently and are almost always detected by the patient. The earlier they are found and treated, the better. Most of the approximately five thousand testicular tumors diagnosed each year occur before age forty, but about a quarter of these tumors occur after that age. Consequently, self-examination every month is recommended until age sixty. I would emphasize that testicular lumps are often benign, but every self-detected lump must be examined by a physician and a decision made about whether it should be removed or biopsied.

Weight Control Overweight by 20 percent or more is a risk factor for uterine cancer, so women should monitor their weight not only in regard to heart disease, but also uterine cancer. As far as I am concerned, that is the only cancer for which, based on consistent and convergent data, overweight is a demonstrated risk factor.

In addition to the above components of the Health-Full-Life Program—all of which relate to heart disease, cancer, or stroke and which compose eleven points of our program—we feel equally important to healthy living are the remaining six categories.

Glaucoma

Each person over age thirty-five should have eye tension and visual fields checked for glaucoma every five years; if the tension is elevated or the visual fields are abnormal, the person should be under the care of an eye doctor.

Glaucoma can be considered hypertension of the eye. When pressure within the eye increases, the result may be eye discomfort and, in many cases, constriction of vision and even blindness. You cannot prevent the increase in tension within the eye, but you can usually control the progression of the accompanying changes by medicating with eyedrops. By so doing, you markedly reduce the likelihood of severe loss of vision. Early detection can be achieved by a simple, painless test.

If the tension is elevated, then it should be followed closely at yearly intervals (or more frequently) and careful assessment should periodically be made of visual fields so it can be determined when medication should be given. I do not mean to suggest that all increased eye tension results in loss of vision. Many people have increased tension but never develop frank glaucoma and visual loss. Nevertheless, if you take 100 persons with increased tension and compare them with 100 persons the same age with normal tension, there is a much greater likelihood of glaucoma with visual loss in the former group.

In the past, many experts have felt that detecting elevated eye tension really made no difference in the long run, but now the treatment of glaucoma is more sophisticated and effective and there are increasing treatment alternatives that include both drugs and lasers. Since treatment is in general more effective, that is all the more reason to check eye tension and refer anyone with an elevated tension for surveillance by an ophthalmologist. If the tension is normal, an individual could still develop glaucoma in the next five years, but that would be very unlikely and, for the most part, a person with a normal eye tension does not have to be checked more frequently than every five years.

Anemia

Each person between the ages of twenty and sixty should have the hemoglobin level determined to detect anemia at least every two years. Once an individual reaches age sixty, the hemoglobin should be tested yearly.

Anemia can be measured in three ways. The number of red blood cells per cubic millimeter of blood can be counted directly under the microscope. A second technique is to measure the amount of hemoglobin in the red blood cells. Hemoglobin, a protein, is the major constituent of the red blood cell and is responsible for the ability of red blood cells to transport oxygen from the lungs to the various body tissues. It is measured as grams per 100 cubic centimeters of blood. The third way is to spin a sample of blood in a centrifuge so that the red cells are all packed together and separated from the plasma, the liquid in which they circulate in the body. The red cell mass, called the hematocrit, is then reported as a percentage of the total blood volume. The most frequently used of the three determinations is the hemoglobin.

Why should anemia be of concern? There are in most instances one of four explanations for the anemia. One is blood loss in a woman due to very heavy menstrual flow. A second is loss of blood from bleeding in the intestinal tract due to diseases such as ulcer or a tumor of the bowel. A third is a poor diet with inadequate intake of iron, which is essential for red blood cell development. The fourth is a deficient intake of vitamins, in particular folic acid, which is needed for the development of red blood cells.

Anemia, which can occur at any age, can be detected readily by examining blood taken by finger prick or from a vein. If the anemia and any feelings of weakness or lassitude are due to dietary lack of iron, dietary lack of folic acid, or blood loss due to heavy menstrual flow, administration of iron or folic acid is all that is needed. Eliminating the anemia may make a great difference in the way the person feels mentally and physically.

Low Back Pain

Low back pain is one of the most frequent causes of absenteeism from work. The figures are staggering. It is said that eight out of ten adults will suffer from low back pain sometime in their lives and that millions of workers are afflicted each year with a yearly economic loss in the $30 billion range. Some low back pain is not preventable, but much of it is, and all that is required is about ten minutes each day of back exercises, preferably each morning; or better still, once in the morning and once in the evening. I would recommend six exercises, each with ten repetitions. Diagrams follow and include: the pelvic tilt, single knee pull toward chest, single leg raise to full extension with the other knee bent, double knee pull toward the chest, stomach-muscle strengthener, and sit-ups with knees bent. It is important to note that when doing the single knee pull and straight leg raising and stomach-tightening exercises, the knee of the leg not being exercised is bent; when doing sit-ups, both knees are bent.

The pelvic tilt is achieved while lying flat on your back on a firm surface by simultaneously tightening the stomach muscles and pushing the buttocks together, thereby flattening out the normal arch in the lower back. Once achieved, the pelvic

LOW BACK EXERCISES

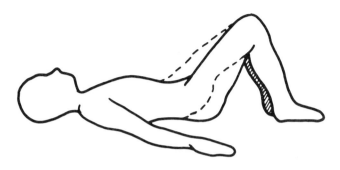

1
Pelvic Tilt
Lie on your back with knees bent. Push the lower part of your back into the floor by tightening your abdominal and buttock muscles, rotating the pelvis upward without bringing your back off the floor. Hold for count of five. Repeat ten times.

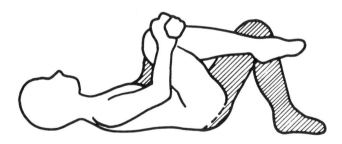

2
Knee Pull
Lie on your back with knees bent. Place feet flat on the floor, tilt pelvis upward as in illustration 1. Take your right knee and pull it toward your chest, hold for count of five. Repeat ten times. Take your left knee and do the same.

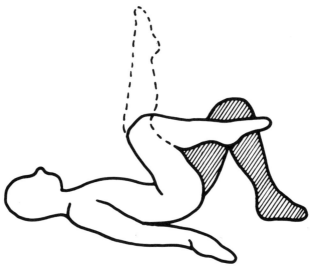

3
Single Leg Raise

Lie on your back with knees bent, feet flat on the floor. Tilt
pelvis upward as in illustration 1. Draw one leg to your chest,
extend as fully as possible, and hold for count of five. Repeat
ten times with each leg.

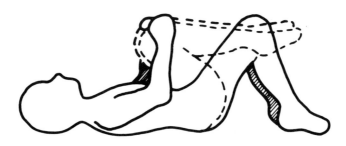

4
Double Knee Pull

Lie on your back with knees bent. Tilt pelvis as in illustration
1; with your hands, pull both knees up to your chest. Hold for
count of five. Repeat ten times.

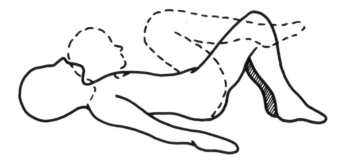

5
Stomach-Muscle Strengthener

Lie on your back, arms resting comfortably at your sides, with knees bent. Bend left leg and draw knee toward head; at the same time, bring head up and forward toward the flexed knee. Stomach muscles will tighten. Hold for count of five. Repeat ten times, then do again with right knee.

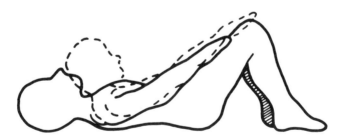

6
Sit-up

Start with your knees bent. Place your arms on your thighs. Tighten your stomach and buttocks, slowly raise head, neck, and shoulders to sitting position and extend your hands to your knees. Hold for count of five. Repeat ten times.

tilt should be held for a count initially of five and then, after you have acclimated yourself to the exercises, to a count of ten.

For the next three exercises, the pelvic tilt should be done as the first part of the exercise so the lower back is flat against the floor or rug, not arched.

The single knee pull consists of bending both knees and pulling one toward your head, using both hands (keeping the other knee bent). Hold for a count of five and then, as with the pelvic tilt, when accustomed to the exercise, to a count of ten. Do ten repetitions with each knee, always keeping the knee not being pulled in a flexed position.

Straight leg raising is done with both knees bent. Do a pelvic tilt, then extend the left leg until it is reasonably straight. Hold as above for a count of five (subsequently work up to a count of ten). Do ten repetitions with each leg.

The double knee pull is a very important exercise. The knees are bent, pelvic tilt achieved, and with one hand on each knee, both knees are brought toward the head, rocking the lower and midback on the floor or rug. You can feel the back flatten; it has no other alternative. Hold for a count of five (subsequently work up to a count of ten), and do ten repetitions.

The fifth exercise will strengthen stomach muscles, an essential ingredient of a strong back. You lie flat on your back, arms at your side or spread out, knees bent, and bring the left knee up toward your head as far as you can; at the same time, you lift your head to bring your chin as far toward that knee as possible. Hold at first for a count of five and, after that is done easily, gradually increase until you are holding for a count of ten. You will feel the effect on your stomach muscles. Then relax and repeat, gradually increasing the number of repetitions to ten. Do the same with the right knee. This exercise does not start with a pelvic tilt.

Sit-ups are done with the legs free (do not hook the feet under a chair or bed). The knees should be bent and stay bent. Pelvic tilt is achieved, then bring the back upright and bend a little forward. Do five sit-ups at first, increasing gradually until the ten-sit-up goal is reached.

Everybody should do low back pain prevention exercises every day. Before undertaking the exercises, loosening up (stretching exercises) should be done. If you are having low back pain now, these exercises should not be performed until you have seen a physician or, in the case of mild pain, until the pain has subsided.

For most people, a few minutes a day of these exercises carried out when you are having no trouble with your back will prevent a lot of avoidable pain and anguish. Of course, it is equally important to sit up with the back supported when sitting in a chair or driving and to bend your knees when picking up objects. And if you are sitting on a soft surface—a bed or chair cushion, for example—when you stand up, use your arms to push off so you are not putting all the pressure on your lower back. You can also do a pelvic tilt (stomach tightened, buttock tightened) literally hundreds of times a day when sitting or standing. Nobody will even notice you are doing this helpful and simple back exercise. I cannot predict with certainty what percentage of low back pain can be avoided, but I know that it is significant. My own experience is instructive.

At age fifteen, I injured my back during wrestling practice. In college, I played at a varsity level and continued to play competitive sports (rugby until age forty-five, squash until the present) at a reasonably high level of proficiency. All that time, I had intermittent back pain, often playing with a supporting brace. As I grew older, it got worse. On lecture tours, I would often be in agony. About seven years ago, I gave two one-hour lectures as part of a medical seminar—a seminar I attended with an extremely painful back. It was excruciating just getting dressed and the lectures themselves were an ordeal, as I stood in a grotesque position, suffering such pain that perspiration poured down my face. One of my colleagues at the seminar was amazed to discover that I did no preventive exercises. He said he had for years experienced similar pain and that low back exercises has changed his life. After my pain subsided, I started to do the exercises outlined in the diagrams that accompany this chapter. They have changed *my* life. I had been ready to give up squash competition. Now I play squash and tennis without a brace and have had no significant problems. But I know I have to sit correctly, bend correctly, support my back by pushing off cushions and beds with my arms, and, above all, I must do those exercises every single day. These simple exercises urged upon me by my colleague represent the most useful medical advice I have ever been given. And so I urge you to spend a few minutes a day to try to prevent low back pain. It will not guarantee that you will never have low back pain, but it offers the potential for avoiding the kind of pain that plagued me for thirty-five years.

Some urge more elaborate exercises. That, of course, means a much greater time commitment. I have found that if too many are recommended and too much time is required, most people end up doing none at all. I believe the six I have suggested will suffice and the time commitment required is quite reasonable. Those inclined to do more should consult some of the books on back pain, their own physicians or an orthopedic (or osteopathic) expert.

Seat Belts

Every person in a moving vehicle should be wearing proper restraints and car doors should be locked.

The evidence is so impressive that it is fair to say that anyone not using proper restraints is a fool. In 1984, almost thirty thousand occupants of vehicles (motorcycles included) were killed in accidents in the United States. Deaths from motor vehicle accidents are the fourth leading cause of death in the United States and by far the leading cause of death among those five to twenty-four years old. The best analysis of the efficacy of seat belts was published in the December 30, 1988, issue of the *Journal of the American Medical Association* by Dr. Elizabeth Mueller Orsay and her colleagues from Chicago. The study, entitled "Prospective Study of the Effect of Safety Belts on Morbidity and Health Care Costs in Motor Vehicle Accidents" was carried out at four Chicago area hospitals, and analyzed 1,364 drivers and passengers who were seen in the hospital emergency units for injuries sustained in motor vehicle accidents. Of these accident victims, 791 (58 percent) used seat belts, whereas 573 (42 percent) did not. They focused particularly on three issues: the severity of the injury, need for hospitalization, and the monetary costs of the injury. The results were dramatic. Those using seat belts showed a:

- 60 percent reduction in the severity of injury;
- 65 percent reduction in the need for hospitalization;
- 66 percent reduction in overall hospital costs.

There were five deaths among the 1,314 injured; all were non-seat-belt users. Safety belt users were better off in frontal, rear, and side collisions. Of the most seriously injured, 82 percent were not using seat belts.

Yet a survey published in the *Journal of the American Medical Association* showed that in the period 1981–83, 75 percent of adult Americans never used seat belts or used them only some of the time. Among the eighteen- to twenty-four-year age group, the nonuse figure was 81 percent, a particularly depressing figure, considering that almost 40 percent of the deaths occur among persons less than twenty-five years of age. A 1985 survey of twenty-one states by the Centers for Disease Control showed that in thirteen of the twenty-one states, more than 60 percent of those surveyed did not use seat belts; in only two states was the percentage of regular seat belt use over 50 percent.

Buckling up is good preventive medicine. About half of all severe auto crashes are frontal crashes, and it is in this type of crash that seat belts are most effective. In side crashes and rollover crashes, a major risk is ejection from the car. That is why, in addition to using seat belts, doors should be locked— an extra precaution against being thrown out of the car after a crash. Proper use of seat belts will reduce deaths or severe injuries to motor vehicle occupants by 60 to 75 percent.

Every state has mandatory restraint laws for those under four years old. You would think that all parents would insist their children be properly restrained, but the figure of restraint usage for the under-four category is no better than 40 percent, a terrible record.

For older children and adults, there are several types of restraints or protection: lap belts, shoulder harnesses, three-point shoulder and lap belts, and air bags. Lap belts or shoulder harnesses by themselves are inadequate. Air bags are useful only in frontal and rear impact crashes; they do not help in side or rollover crashes. So if you have air bags, you still need seat belts. The best protection is the three-point shoulder and lap belts. Air bags, according to a variety of studies, provide added protection, but the increment in protection is at most modest. My own feeling is that no new car should be permitted to be sold in the United States after 1990 unless such three-point restraints are included for both front- and back-seat passengers. Recent government edicts suggest this is likely to happen.

Mandatory use of seat belts does work. In Victoria, Australia, such a law increased seat belt usage from 64 to 75 percent and fatal vehicle accidents in urban areas fell 21 percent. In England, after seat belt laws went into effect, admissions to hospitals from motor vehicle collisions fell 25 percent. At this writing, thirty-three states plus the District of Columbia have implemented mandatory seat belt laws. They vary somewhat from each other, but in my judgment, there are problems with all of them.

For example, only those in the front seat are required to buckle up; the fines for nonuse are so small that the laws will inevitably be ignored by many automobile occupants; and the provisions for police surveillance are often inadequate. So far, after mandatory seat belt laws have been enacted, use has increased dramatically, but within a year the percentage of users usually falls substantially.

Many people oppose air bags or mandatory seat belt use on the grounds that such safety features should be optional. According to this argument, the individual should make a voluntary judgment so long as all he or she risks is his or her own life. That is, to me, a silly argument. We all pay for the $40 billion to $50 billion in yearly health costs from automobile accidents, as these costs are reflected in all our health insurance policies.

There are those who insist, "I don't need seat belts because I am a careful driver." That is ludicrous. Who will guarantee that the other people on the highway are all safe drivers? And no amount of caution can protect against losing control on a wet or icy road.

And it seems to me astounding that with what we know about seat belts, a person will get into a taxicab with a driver he or she does not know and thus be exposed to the possibility of a serious accident in an automobile without functioning seat belts. The lack of seat belts in school buses is equally unconscionable. It ought to be mandatory for every taxicab and every bus to have working seat belts available for every passenger.

It is important to make sure the seat belt is properly attached and is not twisted. This applies particularly to lap belts, which often are twisted and then are fastened. If they remain twisted and there is an accident, the twisted belt might produce rather than prevent injury. It is a simple matter to untwist it and put it on properly. Pregnant women should wear belts in the normal position—the pressure will not have any adverse effect on the baby.

The risk of serious accident for those using motorcycles is very substantial, yet many such riders oppose safety helmets. That is moronic. When mandatory helmet laws were enacted in various states for motorcycle users, the death rates, according to several studies, fell by one-third to about one-half; in those states that repealed the compulsory helmet law, fatality rates rose to 27 to 38 percent more than in states that retained the laws. Studies of motorcycle riders indicate that only 40 to 50 percent would voluntarily wear helmets, but with firm laws actually in place over 90 percent do. Since, in the long run, the expenses of severe injury, prolonged hospitalization, and chronic care are borne by all of us, we are being asked to subsidize the stupidity of motorcycle riders who don't want to wear helmets.

An excellent article in the May 25, 1989, issue of the *New England Journal of Medicine,* by Robert S. Thompson, M.D., and his colleagues from the Group Health Cooperative of Puget Sound, makes a strong case for use of helmets by bicyclists. They studied bicycle injuries and found that wearing helmets reduced the risk of serious head injury by 85 percent.

There is one additional approach that will help persuade drivers and passengers to use restraints. We should have a tough policy permitting a 50 percent reduction in injury payments to those who fail to use restraints. After all, if they failed to use a seat belt, the severity of an injury is partly their fault. I would also favor potential suspension of a driving license after three convictions for failure to use seat belts, and the driver should be held responsible for each passenger. If they won't buckle up, they should not be permitted to ride in the car.

The experience with the seat belt law in Massachusetts is both instructive and discouraging. The Massachusetts law, like that of most states, was weak when it was passed in 1986; violation resulted in a maximum fine of only $15. After the law was passed, a careful study by investigators at Boston University School of Public Health indicated that seat belt use increased from 20 to 37 percent among adults. Those complying with the new law were, for the most part, the safest drivers; the drug users, those repeatedly ticketed for speeding, those with a history of ignoring red lights, the alcohol abusers, did not comply with the new law. Even the majority of those who said they believed seat belt laws reduced injury and death did not comply. Then the campaign for repeal started; the opponents noted that car occupant deaths fell only 1 percent when the law was in force, but they overlooked the fact that occupant deaths rose 4 percent in other New England states during the same period. And, of course, the most dangerous drivers ignored the law.

Now the law is repealed and seat belt use is down to 24 percent among adults. At this writing, eleven other states are considering repeal of compulsory seat belt laws. That is just plain stupid.

The evidence now clearly shows that if laws are to be effective:

- They must have substantial penalties (fines) for nonobservance;
- The police must be able to stop and ticket people if seat belts are not being used. In many states the police can stop a car only for some other offense (such as speeding) and then specifically charge the occupants with seat belt law violation if, in addition to the primary offense, there is evidence of nonuse of seat belts for front seat occupants;
- There must be reduction in personal injury payments by insurance companies if injured occupants were not using seat belts.

Immunization

Effective vaccines are available for measles, mumps, and German measles. A vaccine for chicken pox is available, but its efficacy is less certain and at present it is not recommended for general use. The vaccines for measles, mumps, and German measles are living, weakened viruses that probably confer lifelong protection. They should be given during the first few years of life, but if it is necessary that they be given during the first year (when the response of the infant may be less than desirable), they should be given again before the child is six years old. Table 9 shows a recommended schedule for immunizations.

It is distressing to realize that there still are millions of school-age children who have not been vaccinated against these viruses. It is true that the vaccines have some side effects, including, rarely, brain inflammation or encephalitis. This occurs, for example, approximately once for every 1 million doses of measles vaccine, but the consequences of the natural infection are far worse.

TABLE 9

Recommended Immunizations

Immunization	Age
Measles Mumps	Between ages one and four. A measles booster is recommended at about age twelve.
German measles	Ideally, at eleven or twelve (especially for girls), but often given with measles and mumps.
Diphtheria Pertussis (whooping cough) Tetanus	Three times during first year, then two times between one and one-half and six years; thereafter, tetanus every ten years.
Polio (oral)	Two to three times during first year, then at fifteen to eighteen months, and again at age five to six; after age twenty, one booster. Adults immunized for first time should be given killed vaccine by injection.
Smallpox	Not needed.
Influenza	Recommended yearly for adults over sixty and for those with chronic lung or heart disease; during epidemics, recommended for everyone.
Typhoid	Not needed.
Pneumonia	Recommended for adults suffering from chronic lung disease or heart failure with congestion, alcoholics, those in nursing homes or institutions for mentally or physically disabled, those suffering from sickle cell anemia; those who have had their spleen removed; probably should be given to all persons over age sixty.
Hepatitis B	Recommended at present for certain health care workers, certain patients such as those undergoing dialysis, those traveling to areas of the world where there is a lot of hepatitis B.

Mumps can produce deafness, inflammation of the pancreas, brain inflammation, arthritis, and, in young men after puberty, painful testicular swelling and inflammation. The latter usually involves only one testicle and does not usually produce sterility, but cases of sterility have been reported.

There is a vaccine that combines all three viruses—mumps, measles, and German measles. It can be given once by injection in the arm between ages one and four (usually at fifteen months), and it appears to confer lifelong protection.

The vaccines have been available only since the 1960s; consequently, the duration of protection is not yet absolutely clear, but the evidence thus far is that only one injection need be given. Actually, for German measles, the ideal would be to give each girl a German measles vaccination at age twelve to guard against the possibility the vaccine will lose its protective power in twenty years. This is unlikely, but it will be another decade or so before we can be sure. Conceivably, those injected at ages one to three could be susceptible again at age twenty-three; this would be highly undesirable since the major danger of German measles is infection early in pregnancy. If girls were immunized at age twelve and the vaccine did happen to lose effectiveness twenty years later, they would be protected until their early thirties, and many at that age would already have given birth to all the children they planned to have. Presumably, however, protection is long-lasting and vaccination at ages one to three will confer permanent protection.

An encouraging study in this regard was published in the *Journal of the American Medical Association* of June 3, 1988, by Susan Chu, Ph.D., and her colleagues. They found that more than 90 percent of children given rubella vaccine showed evidence of persisting protection sixteen years later. Still, the most conservative recommendation would be mumps and measles vaccine at ages one to four, and German measles (rubella) vaccine at age twelve. This is what is done in some countries in Europe, but most experts in the United States believe it is best to get everybody protected in the first few years of life.

I should point out that thanks to a determined drive led by the Centers for Disease Control, the progress against measles has been phenomenal. This is due in large part to regulations compelling vaccination prior to matriculation in grade school. In the 1960s and early 1970s, there were about 500,000 cases per year; now there are only a few thousand, though unexpected small epidemics still occur. Even with those small epidemics, the total number of cases for each year is well under 10,000.

If a woman of childbearing age who might become pregnant has not received rubella vaccine, she should have a blood test for rubella antibodies. If antibody signifying past infection is not present, she should be immunized before getting pregnant, or if pregnant, rubella vaccine should be given shortly after delivery. Vaccine should not be given to any woman who plans to get pregnant in the next three months. If a woman was immunized as a child, it still makes sense before getting pregnant to obtain a blood test to be sure the protection persists. If the blood test does not show continuing immunity, another vaccination should be given. Unfortunately, adverse reactions can occur; usually these are mild, consisting of transient joint discomfort, but, in a few cases, prolonged nervous system and joint abnormalities have occurred. Fortunately, the number of women suffering serious complications is very small.

The recommendation for diphtheria vaccine is every ten years throughout adulthood after primary immunization as a child. My own feeling is somewhat different. There is very little diphtheria in the country, and those cases that are reported are for the most part confined to special subpopulations in which the children have not been immunized. Consequently, I do not recommend diphtheria immunization for adult members of my family and consider it optional for the general adult population. As far as I am concerned, once adulthood is reached, no diphtheria immunization is needed unless it becomes a problem in your community. Others argue that diphtheria should be given because the individual might travel to underdeveloped areas of the world where diphtheria is a problem, and diphtheria vaccine can be given in the same injection as tetanus. I continue to believe it should be optional.

Tetanus is given along with diphtheria and whooping cough immunization in the first six years of life. Thereafter, the recommendation is reimmunization with tetanus toxoid once every ten years. I strongly concur with that recommendation. It should be a part of your health calendar. It might help to remember it if you automatically get a tetanus shot at the beginning of each decade: age twenty, thirty, forty, etc. There are only one hundred to two hundred cases reported each year in the United States (probably this is a falsely low figure because of underreporting), but tetanus is a fearsome disease with a high mortality rate. Older persons may respond less well to the vaccine, and those over age sixty should probably get a booster every five years.

Poliomyelitis is the paradigm of a successful immunization program against a terrible disease. In the 1950s, there were thousands of cases of paralytic disease every year. After the development of the Salk vaccine, consisting of killed polio organisms, and the Sabin oral live-polio vaccine, the number of cases fell dramatically so that now there are fewer than twenty cases each year in the United States. The present recommendation is two or three doses of the oral vaccine in the first year of life, followed by boosters at fifteen months and again at five to six years.

A bitter fight has arisen between the advocates of the oral live vaccine and the killed injected vaccine. Of the few cases of paralytic polio in the United States each year, about half arise from the vaccine itself, paralysis occurring either in the person getting the vaccine or in someone who has direct contact with that person. This is a very low complication rate, considering the millions of doses of vaccine administered each year, but it has served to ignite the smoldering debate between the proponents of the Sabin live vaccine and those of the Salk killed vaccine. It is not a critical debate from the public health point of view. If all of the ten to twenty cases per year of paralysis were caused by the Sabin oral vaccine, the accomplishments of the vaccine would still be considered phenomenal—down from thousands of paralytic cases to ten to twenty, most of which are limited in degree of severity.

The Salk people say you could have the same protection with no risk of paralysis by using killed vaccine, but the problems with the killed vaccine are twofold. First, not all killed vaccines are as effective as the oral vaccine, and, second, the oral live vaccine clearly provides protection for a much longer period of time. Those receiving the killed vaccine by injection must be revaccinated every few years, which is likely to reduce the compliance rate and, by so doing, increase the pool of nonimmunized persons.

Because the live oral polio vaccine is so effective, provides such prolonged protection, and can even provide protection for the nonvaccinated, I believe we should continue to use it, even though there is a tiny risk of inducing polio (about one case per 3 million to 5 million doses).

At present, the vaccine containing all three polio-type viruses is given at two, four, and six months (or alternatively only at two of those times) and a booster dose is given a year later. The same general schedule is used for initial vaccination with the killed vaccine. Because nobody knows whether live vaccine protection lasts for life, I recommend a single booster dose of vaccine as an adult. The risk of paralysis from the live vaccine in previously immunized persons is virtually nil. If anyone in the household has an underlying disease that results in defects in immunity, the adult booster dose of live virus should not be given, since the virus can spread from the vaccinee and threaten persons with such immune defects. Even though the risk is tiny, this is such a thorny problem that the Scientific Advisory Board of Health-Full-Life has decided that all adult booster injections should be with the Salk killed vaccine. For most people, only a single booster need be given during adulthood. Many experts, including some members of our Scientific Advisory Board, believe that live polio vaccine immunity is lifelong and therefore no adult booster is needed, except for those traveling to areas of the world where polio is rampant. I personally advocate a single adult booster using the killed vaccine and would give additional boosters only for those traveling to polio-infected areas if they have not had a killed vaccine booster in the last ten years. If someone has been given a booster with live polio vaccine as an adult, no additional booster is ever needed.

It is estimated that 30 percent of adults were either never immunized or received inadequate immunization. That presents a special problem. The risk of paralysis is higher in adults who have never been immunized and take the oral live vaccine. For such adults, immunization should be with the killed vaccine, which may require a booster every five years. Adults whose children are being immunized with oral vaccine are at risk if they have never been immunized because they can catch the live virus from their children; they should receive the killed vaccine (three injections) before their children receive the live vaccine.

It still makes sense to have influenza immunization whenever the evidence is clear that a major epidemic is on its way. For those over age twenty-five, a single injection will do; for those aged thirteen to twenty-five, two injections may be necessary. Immunization is ordinarily not necessary for those under age thirteen since they rarely develop severe complications. Those over age sixty and those with significant heart or lung disease (such as rheumatic heart disease or emphysema) should have an injection every fall. The adverse neurological effects (paralysis) from influenza vaccine that occurred after use of the swine flu vaccine in 1977–78 have not been observed since, and there is no reason to expect a recurrence of that episode.

Recently, a vaccine has been developed for one of the most important causes of pneumonia, the pneumococcus bacterium. The question is how effective is the vaccine and who should take it. We do not yet have adequate answers, but it would appear that anyone who is inordinately susceptible to infection with this organism should take the vaccine. This would include those who have chronic lung disease associated with infection (such as chronic bronchitis), those who have had their spleen removed, those who suffer from sickle cell anemia, and those over age sixty.

Interestingly, the vaccine has been advocated for those with chronic heart disease, diabetes, and kidney failure, but none of these groups has increased susceptibility to infection with the pneumococcus organism and, consequently, I do not advocate the vaccine for such persons. If a person has lung congestion as a result of heart disease, the vaccine is recommended. Additionally, those in nursing homes or other chronic-care facilities should be vaccinated, since pneumococcal infections are frequent in such places. Alcoholics are also extraordinarily susceptible to pneumococcal infections and should be vaccinated. Unfortunately, there is at present a continuing controversy over the effectiveness of the pneumococcus vaccine, different studies showing it to have a 0 to 70 percent effectiveness. I believe that, pending additional data, it is indicated for the groups listed in table 9. However, I should again emphasize that we do not have all the answers and some studies do not support the use of the vaccine routinely for older persons.

Hepatitis is a virus infection of the liver that can be mild, severe, or even lethal. There are three major types, known as A, B, and non-A, non-B. Hepatitis A grows in the intestinal tract and can be transmitted from person to person through close contact or by contaminated water or food. B circulates in the blood and can be transmitted via saliva, semen, and other body fluids. Non-A, non-B is also transmitted by blood. The B virus can get in through any abrasion. If, for example, the saliva from a person with hepatitis B gets on the hand of a friend or relative who has a cut on that hand, the friend or relative can contract hepatitis. A dentist with hepatitis B can give it to his patients and infrequently a man can transmit it to a woman during intercourse.

If a person develops hepatitis A, the most obvious manifestation is yellowing of the eyes and darkening of the color of the urine. This occurs in most cases two to six weeks after exposure. That two- to six-week period is called the "incubation period"; a person with hepatitis is contagious for two weeks before the jaundice appears and for one week afterward.

Hepatitis A can be prevented by a single injection of gamma globulin. The question, then, is who should get it. The answer: those persons in close contact with the patient during that two- to six-week period. For the most part, that would be limited to household contacts—not casual contacts —office co-workers, and other close companions. If an epidemic seems likely as a consequence of exposure to a common source, such as contaminated water or food, then theoretically, as soon as the first few cases are discovered, the rest of those exposed should receive gamma globulin, a blood-derived substance that contains antibodies that help control the hepatitis virus. In actual practice, though, by the time the possibility of an epidemic is recognized, it is too late for gamma globulin to help. Once a person has had hepatitis A, there is lifelong protection against reinfection; if that person is exposed again to hepatitis A, no gamma globulin is needed. In the near future, a vaccine will be available for hepatitis A.

Hepatitis B is a more severe disease. It is usually acquired through transfusions, accidental needle penetrations with contaminated blood, or occasionally by very close contact with an individual sick with the disease. Drug addicts taking heroin and other drugs by needle, and homosexual men, frequently get hepatitis B. There is a special form of gamma globulin that is effective in preventing this disease, but it is expensive and should be reserved for individuals who have accidentally stuck themselves with needles or otherwise contaminated themselves with the blood of a person with hepatitis B. For others who have close contact with a person with hepatitis B, regular gamma globulin will suffice.

There are two vaccines, one using treated live virus and a new genetically engineered vaccine using a gene from the hepatitis B virus that is put into a yeast cell; material is then harvested that can be used for immunization. The genetically engineered vaccine is not a complete virus and it is the preferred vaccine. It is recommended for many health care workers exposed to blood or blood products and for those who will be traveling to areas of the world with a lot of hepatitis B. I would suspect it will also be advocated for those with kidney failure undergoing hemodialysis, and for intravenous drug abusers and homosexuals.

Osteoporosis

Both men and women should be sure their calcium intake is adequate. Osteoporosis—bone thinning—is a frequently incapacitating and sometimes life-threatening disease. According to the National Institutes of Health Consensus Conference, published August 10, 1984, in the *Journal of the American Medical Association,* there are about 1.3 million fractures each year in the United States attributable to osteoporosis (most of these occur in women over fifty). One out of every six women living to an old age will suffer a hip fracture due at least in part to osteoporosis. There are about 200,000 hip fractures each year; of those who sustain such fractures, at least 20 percent will die in the next three months as a result of being bedridden and other complications. For those who survive, the hip fracture often results in permanent disability, chronic pain, and increased dependency on other people. Half the women over seventy-five have had fractures of the spine due to osteoporosis; these so-called compression fractures can result in the "dwindling" syndrome; that is, the women actually become smaller as the spinal skeleton compresses because of the fractures.

The economic cost of osteoporosis, which affects at least 15 million Americans, according to an excellent review by Dr. Steven R. Cummings and his colleagues published in 1985 in *Epidemiologic Reviews,* is at least $6 billion a year. The number of people involved and the costs can only become greater as the number of persons over the age of sixty-five in the United States increases from the present 30 million to about 50 million by the year 2030.

Bone strength is dependent on its calcium content. Bone mass builds during adolescence and reaches a peak between ages twenty and forty, usually between thirty and thirty-seven. At peak, bone density is greater in men than in women and greater in blacks than in whites. There are several studies showing that peak bone density can be related to calcium intake patterns during the previous twenty years. That is an important observation because the evidence is that the majority of Americans do not have an adequate calcium intake. However, not all studies on the simple relationship of calcium intake to peak bone density or mass show a strong positive correlation.

After age forty or forty-five, there is normally bone density loss that amounts to about 1 percent per year. Since white women start with a smaller bone mass, they are most susceptible to the effects of bone loss, which is accelerated during the first five to ten years after menopause. The loss makes white women particularly prone to wrist, spine, and hip fractures; the spine fractures occur mostly between ages fifty and seventy and the hip fractures after age sixty-five.

What can be done to prevent this? There is much about osteoporosis that is not clear, but surely everyone should pay attention to calcium intake. In the past, the recommendation called for a daily intake of 800 milligrams of calcium. That is now being changed to 1,000 milligrams a day. Most women take in less than 500 milligrams a day. Health-Full-Life recommends that every male adult include 1,000 milligrams of calcium in the diet and every female ingest 1,200 to 1,500 milligrams a day; after menopause, the daily calcium intake should certainly be increased to 1,500 milligrams a day. Although we advocate increasing the calcium intake to prevent osteoporosis, I should emphasize that although this may potentially prevent osteoporosis, we don't have the data to be sure. The data suggesting that calcium intake in early and teenage life is important in determining bone strength are reasonably good, but the evidence that increasing calcium intake in women during the first five to ten years after the menopause prevents subsequent osteoporosis and bone fractures is far less secure.

Indeed, a most careful study by Dr. Bente Riis and his colleagues from the University of Copenhagen in Denmark was published in January 1987 in the *New England Journal of Medicine*. They gave a very small group of postmenopausal women two grams a day of calcium carbonate, did sophisticated and detailed measurements over a two-year study and found that the calcium supplement produced only a small reduction in bone loss compared to controls. They concluded that calcium supplements given to postmenopausal women are not very helpful in preventing the bone loss that leads to osteoporosis and bone fractures. This study did not exclude the possibility that certain types of calcium intake they did not study could have helped prevent osteoporosis. There are now several other good studies supporting the notion that increasing calcium in the diet after the menopause or giving calcium supplements will not significantly reduce the risk of osteoporosis and subsequent bone fractures. So making sure calcium intake is adequate makes sense particularly for young women, but it is no panacea, especially for those who are postmenopausal.

There is increasing emphasis on regular exercise during adolescent and premenopause adult years as a mechanism for achieving a greater peak bone mass and density. Similarly, it is suggested that regular exercise after menopause will slow bone loss. Neither idea is adequately documented. Although several studies support the association between intensity of exercise and peak bone strength, many more data are needed before a definitive judgment can be made. The same is true of slowing bone loss after age forty-five by regular exercise. Some studies support the notion, but others do not. Even if exercise is effective, we don't know how much or what kind.

There is increasing interest in measuring bone density in the high-risk group, white women over age forty-five. The problems with such measurements are several. First, there is a debate about what to measure. There are two types of bone, cortical and trabecular. Overall, about 80 percent of body bone is cortical, but the spinal column is mostly trabecular. The question is how to do one measurement that simultaneously predicts fractures of the hip, forearm, and spine. Some experts urge sophisticated and expensive X-ray studies of the spine and hip. Others favor special X ray—like studies of the forearm or of the foot. The least expensive technique involves an X ray of the hand that is processed by computer, but there is a lot of dispute about its accuracy and predictive value.

Unfortunately, we do not know exactly how well the tests predict the likelihood of spine or hip fractures, and each test is likely to cost between $50 and $200. We need a reliable test because there are essentially two types of women, those who lose the usual 1 percent per year after menopause and a much smaller number of women who lose bone density very rapidly after menopause. For the former group, making sure their calcium intake is adequate, and urging regular exercise, may be enough, but the latter group probably needs treatment with estrogens. At present, estrogen administration is the most effective approach to stopping postmenopausal bone loss.

At its June 1986 meeting, the Scientific Advisory Board of Health-Full-Life decided that no test of bone density or bone mass was both effective and reasonably inexpensive, so that none could be recommended for routine use on ostensibly healthy postmenopausal women. As soon as a good, reliable, inexpensive test is available, we will embrace it so we can pick out that small percentage of women who are postmenopausal rapid losers and therefore at very high risk for severe bone loss and fractures. But the fact is that the majority of osteoporotic fractures will not come from the small number of women who are rapid losers, but from the much larger group of women who show normal postmenopausal bone loss. And we really do not know how much protection we can offer by increasing calcium intake and by exercise.

Why not, then, give all postmenopausal women estrogens? Multiple studies are now in agreement that estrogen administration starting at the time of menopause or within several years after will strikingly slow bone loss; indeed, in some studies it is completely effective.

One persistent question is whether fractures will actually

be prevented even if estrogens are given and bone loss lessened. There are six solid studies, the most impressive of which was published in the *New England Journal of Medicine* of November 5, 1987, summarizing long-term analysis of 2,873 women in the Framingham program. In this, as in most of the other studies, those women who had used estrogens after menopause were less likely to suffer fractures. We do not yet know the minimum estrogen dose required or how long estrogens must be given. So dogmatic statements about estrogens and osteoporosis or bone fractures are not warranted. If, however, estrogens *are* to be used for preventing bone loss, the dosage should be as small as possible.

Once estrogens are started, the evidence suggests they must be continued for at least ten years. When the estrogens are stopped, bone loss starts again. The argument is that the ten-year delay will postpone bone loss and fractures for so long that many more women will live out their lives without ever suffering such fractures. However, there are several studies showing that after estrogens are stopped, bone loss not only resumes, but its speed may be accelerated.

It is well to remember that estrogens in contraceptive pills were associated with increased risk of clots and strokes in young women, especially those with other risk factors such as high blood pressure or smoking. In older women, there are likely to be more of these risk factors; consequently, estrogens should not be administered promiscuously, and there had better be good epidemiologic surveillance to detect any patterns of adverse effects as soon as possible. I am still concerned that women of fifty-five and older who are given estrogens for a prolonged period may be at increased risk for stroke and clots in the veins even though there is at present no persuasive evidence documenting these fears. Those who recommend that all women receive estrogens starting at the onset of the menopause also point out that the majority of studies suggest that in postmenopausal women, estrogens provide significant protection against coronary heart disease, apparently by increasing blood levels of protective high-density proteins (HDL). However, two studies suggest just the opposite: estrogens increased the risk for either heart attacks or heart pain. There is also a preliminary and not very impressive study suggesting that estrogen administration will actually reduce the likelihood of stroke; here much more data is needed.

We should recall that promiscuous use of estrogens in the 1960s and early 1970s resulted in an increase in cancer of the uterus, and there is still a debate about the aftereffects of estrogen use after the estrogens are stopped. It was thought that after stopping estrogen treatment, the risk of endometrial, or uterine, cancer dropped rapidly. But an article in the *New England Journal of Medicine* of October 17, 1985, by Sam Shapiro, Ph.D., and his colleagues noted that if a woman had used estrogens for a year or longer, her increased risk for uterine cancer remained for at least ten years after discontinuing estrogen treatment.

Those who advocate estrogens in women say the risk of uterine cancer can be reduced markedly by adding progesterone drugs. According to two very good studies, the addition of progesterone drugs does not reduce the beneficial effects of estrogens. However, the estrogen-progesterone combination is no panacea. Women given some estrogen-progesterone combinations will continue to have a bleeding period every month; a lot of women don't want that. If progesterone drugs are added, there may be additional unpleasant reactions; these include depression, anxiety, breast tenderness, backache, abdominal cramps, fluid accumulation, and irritability.

There is also the worry that estrogens may increase the risks of breast and cervical cancer. Most studies on these kinds of cancers show no association with estrogens, but some studies do, especially among those women using estrogens for many years.

Our dilemma, then, is that we have no inexpensive, predictably accurate screening test that will readily identify those women who are fast bone losers, and Health-Full-Life is not yet ready to urge estrogens on all postmenopausal women. These concerns will not stop the doctors from another estrogen-prescribing binge. The public should realize there are no free rides; some people given the estrogens will suffer adverse effects. Whether the harm will clearly be outweighed by the benefits is not yet known. In this book, I intend to be firm in my recommendations, but in this case, regarding the use of postmenopausal estrogens, I have to leave the decision to the woman and her doctor. I have outlined both the potential or documented benefits and the potential or documented risks. Each woman must make the final decision herself.

There may be alternatives to estrogens in the future. A group from Belgium reported in 1987 on a substance called "calcitonin," which is sprayed into the nose five days a week for a year. Postmenopausal women who took calcium alone lost 3 percent of bone density in one year, whereas those who took calcium plus calcitonin actually gained some bone strength. If calcitonin nasal spray can be shown to prevent osteoporosis and fractures, and if it does not produce serious side effects, that would be very exciting. Others believe that fluoride administration will prevent osteoporosis, but there remain a lot of questions both about the effectiveness of fluorides and their toxic effects.

The situation in regard to prevention of osteoporosis is not satisfactory. Adequate calcium intake during adolescence and adult life and exercise are reasonable recommendations at present, but as more research studies become available, the recommendations will almost surely change, particularly in regard to use of estrogens and progestogens.

The program I have outlined above is the minimum necessary and each component can be justified. If you wish to do more because it makes you feel better, there is nothing wrong with that, but you should realize that the evidence for adding other procedures to our program is at best uncertain.

The Health-Full-Life Program does not include some tests and examinations that have been considered virtually obligatory in past decades. These are listed in table 10 together with reasons for their noninclusion. The most notable of these is the general yearly physical examination, which, as

TABLE 10

What We Do Not Do and Why

Test or Examination	Why Not Done
General yearly physical examination	No evidence it is effective in disease prevention. An initial physical examination and then one every decade is adequate. But it is important to look for skin and mouth cancers yearly after age thirty-five.
White blood cell count	Not useful as routine in asymptomatic persons.
Urinalysis	No evidence it makes a difference in an asymptomatic person. However, should be done routinely in pregnant women.
Routine or yearly chest X ray	Not cost-effective in asymptomatic persons. If done at ages twenty, forty, and sixty, that is adequate.
Routine or yearly electrocardiogram	Not cost-effective in asymptomatic persons. It is much better to study the risk factors for heart disease (blood pressure, cholesterol, HDL, weight, smoking). If done at ages twenty, forty, and sixty, that is quite adequate.
Yearly prostate examination after age forty or fifty	This is a poor way of detecting prostate cancer in time to change the outcome.
Routine yearly pelvic examination	A Pap smear is important but the rest of the pelvic examination is not cost-effective in asymptomatic women.

far as I am concerned, is for the most part a waste of time in an apparently healthy adult. Virtually every expert agrees with that assessment, yet most practicing doctors still think that the yearly physical examination is indicated and the public expects it. One thing is sure: a lot of money is being wasted on the yearly physical examination.

A general physical examination every decade is all that is needed in a person with no symptoms. Of course, if a person has specific complaints, a physical examination should be done and the physician should always look for skin or oral lesions that might be cancerous or turn to cancer; and every woman who is thirty years of age or older should have a breast examination by a physician or nurse yearly.

I believe that blood sugar levels should be measured every year and those with high levels (but no symptoms) should be urged to lose weight to try to normalize the values; if that doesn't work, the next step is to urge reduction in dietary sugar intake. But the blood sugar is not listed as one of the core parts of the program because we don't really know whether early detection of a high blood sugar (glucose level) in a person with no symptoms makes any difference in eventual outcome. It has never been clear whether the dreaded eye and vascular complications, including reduced vision, blindness, strokes, and reduction in blood supply to an extremity or the brain, are due to the sugar level itself, to the abnormalities in cholesterol and other fats in the blood, or to some other factor. Some of those at diabetes centers, such as the Joslin Clinic in Boston, are convinced that detecting a blood sugar elevation in a person without any symptoms is useful and that rigid control of the blood sugar will prevent damage to the heart, kidneys, eyes, nervous system, and blood vessels. Nevertheless, at present we do not have convincing evidence to indicate whether it really makes a difference if diabetes is detected when a person has no symptoms compared to waiting until diabetic symptoms appear and then treating vigorously.

It does help to know the glucose level in a person with a high cholesterol level. Both may return to normal with weight loss, but if the cholesterol and glucose levels remain elevated, it may be necessary to try and control the glucose level by dietary reduction of sugar intake or medications in the hope that normalizing the glucose concentration will result in a reduction in cholesterol level. If the blood sugar remains significantly elevated after weight control, careful consideration should be given to possible insulin treatment even if the person has no symptoms.

Can detection of blood in the urine be useful in the early diagnosis of bladder or kidney cancer? If there is bright red blood, it can be helpful. Actually, obvious blood is usually caused by a disease other than cancer, but it must be investigated expeditiously. What about a little bleeding that can be detected only by microscopic examination of the urine or by putting a chemically treated stick into the urine and observing a color change? Nobody knows whether finding slight bleeding by that technique would result in such early detection of bladder or kidney cancer that the survival rate would improve. Unfortunately, if such a test were done routinely, the cost would be enormous, because in the overwhelming majority of cases, an expensive work-up for the slight bleeding would show no disease, or benign disease not requiring any treatment. Since the false positive rate would be very high, and we do not know if it would make any difference in outcome of bladder or kidney cancers, there is no justification for including a test for microscopic blood in the urine in the Health-Full-Life Program.

Almost everything about prostatic cancer remains an enigma. The polar views are, on the one hand, that after age fifty rectal examination for prostatic cancer should be done twice yearly and, on the other hand, that fast-growing prostatic cancers do not respond to treatment anyway and slower-growing tumors may need no treatment even if they are present for five, ten, or twenty years. Interestingly, both of these widely divergent views can be supported by reasonable evidence. The argument that the bigger the tumor, the more likely that the lymph nodes outside the prostate will be involved is probably true, but even if the nodes are involved, the course of the disease is unpredictable and may be very indolent.

About 40 percent of all prostatic cancers are detected when localized. Half of these are found incidentally at surgery or autopsy and are so small they cannot be detected by any screening tests. The other half are called Stage 2 or Stage B. That, in turn, is subdivided into three categories—a small nodule in one part of the prostate gland (B-1), a larger one involving much of one lobe (B-2), and an even larger one involving much of the gland (B-3). There is no evidence that detecting B-2 or B-3 prostate cancers by routine rectal examination makes any difference in the final outcome. Stage B-1 constitutes around 7 percent of all prostate cancers, a percentage that, if detected at this early stage, has a very good outcome if removed or treated by radiation. The problem is that nobody really knows whether that small percentage with B-1 tumors would have done just as well with no treatment or no treatment until symptoms appeared, and it appears that most B-1 cancers are not felt on rectal examination. Dr. Daniel Miller, director of the renowned Strang Clinic in New York City and a world authority on cancer prevention, believes that in the hope of detecting B-1 tumors, men should have a rectal examination every other year from age fifty until age fifty-five, then yearly thereafter. In the Health-Full-Life Program, we will do rectal examinations at the time of left-side colonoscopy (every five years after age forty-five), and once in between colonoscopy examinations after age fifty. There is no need to worry about prostatic cancer prior to age fifty; 99 percent of all prostate cancers occur after that age.

I would emphasize that my views are shared by most experts who have examined this problem. Perhaps the best recent review documenting the inefficiency of the routine rectal examination for prostatic cancer appears in the December 1985 *American Journal of Preventive Medicine,* authored by Dr. Richard Love of the University of Wisconsin Center for Health Sciences.

What about routine urinalysis? It should be done in pregnant women, since silent urinary tract infection can result in adverse pregnancy outcome, including stillbirths and miscarriages. It is also true that while a small number of studies suggest that silent urinary tract infections can result in increased mortality, the overwhelming majority of infectious disease experts believe that there is no evidence that the infection shortens the life of women, who suffer most from these infections. In men, the infection frequently results from obstruction, often by an enlarged prostate gland, and is usually accompanied by symptoms.

Many people feel it important for their own physical and mental well-being to have yearly physicals, X rays, and other examinations, as well as yearly proctoscopies. They need that visit to the physician to give them a feeling of security. It is expensive, and for the most part unnecessary, but if you are willing to accept the costs and it makes you feel better, go to it. After all, psychological health is very important, and much of what the family doctor or internist does is to allay fears. The program I propose consists of what we think is needed and documented; if you wish to do more, that, of course, is your decision. But every adult should follow the basic Health-Full-Life Program. It will totally prevent some diseases, and it will allow such early detection of others that serious harm can be avoided. And it has another marvelous benefit. For those whose tests are normal, the Health-Full-Life Program can provide reassurance and feelings of well-being that can enrich one's life.

2

The Sixty-Plus
Health-Full-Life
Program

The program for those older than sixty is summarized in table 11. For the most part, it does not differ from that for younger persons. Of the seventeen points in the program, only one is dropped entirely; that is testicular examination for cancer, which has a very low incidence after sixty. There has been some suggestion that yearly measurement of blood pressure is not necessary because treatment of high blood pressure in older persons is not effective. This is not true. A study published in the September 13, 1986, issue of *Lancet* showed that treatment of high blood pressure in those over sixty years of age was beneficial, although for those over age eighty no benefit could be demonstrated. This study conducted by the European Working Party on High Blood Pressure in the Elderly is an important study. Even the negative results in the over-eighty group may have to be reconsidered since that group had relatively few participants; it may well be that treatment in the very old will still be found valuable.

For older persons, a different and more extensive health-assessment questionnaire is used, one that also focuses on social supports, disabilities, functional physical capacity, loneliness, and mental functioning. Often the quality of life can be dramatically improved by simple actions in these areas. Several tests are added. These include taste and smell evaluation and more extensive tests for hearing and vision. The reasons for the last two are obvious, and the results can often lead to effective intervention that can dramatically im-

---

TABLE 11

Health-Full-Life for Seniors

Cholesterol and high-density proteins yearly
Hemoglobin and blood sugar yearly
Blood pressure determined yearly
Pap smear every two years
Breast self-examination monthly
Mammography yearly
Stools for blood yearly
Left-side colonoscopy every five years
Testing for taste, smell, hearing, and vision yearly
Glaucoma testing every five years
Evaluation of social support and disabilities yearly
Prostate examination every two to three years
Immunization updating yearly
Low back exercises
Osteoporosis dietary prevention
Smoking elimination or control
Seat belt usage

---

prove the quality of life. A British study found that more than 70 percent of persons over the age of sixty-five had defects in either vision or hearing (or both) that needed correction. For those with failing vision, the interventions can range from change in the prescription for glasses to cataract removal. For those with hearing loss, hearing aids may help immensely.

The approach to decrements in the capacity to taste or smell is much more difficult. A significant percentage of older persons lose taste and smell discrimination either as a "normal" accompaniment to the aging process or as a result of underlying disease. The loss of either can have a very negative effect on the quality of life.

Regular testing of the sensory functions of taste, smell, vision, and hearing is important. Although it is well known that impairment of vision and hearing can adversely affect the quality of life, it is not adequately appreciated that deficits in taste and smell can have an equally devastating effect. Even in our best retirement and nursing home facilities, taste and smell are rarely tested. Impairment of taste and smell is usually selective, not total, but can cause loss of appetite with resultant weight loss and sometimes depression, loss of zest for life, weakness, and even loss of memory and other mental functions. Often a nutritional evaluation can result in a dietary prescription that works around the partial taste and/or smell defects and provides foods that still taste and smell good to the individual; often the quality of life can be changed dramatically for the better. Every facility caring for older persons should regularly test taste, smell, hearing, and vision and take corrective measures, if possible.

It is important not to assume that all or even most fractures in middle-aged and elderly people are related to underlying osteoporosis. For many, the problem is repeated falls; the likelihood of a given fall resulting in fracture is, of course, increased among those suffering from osteoporosis. Obviously, any measures that will prevent fractures, both those due to osteoporosis and those due solely to falls, would be very useful. A fascinating study was published in the *New England Journal of Medicine* on February 14, 1987, by a group of investigators from the Vanderbilt University School of Medicine. They studied 1,021 elderly persons who suffered hip fractures and matched them with appropriate controls. Those taking longer-acting sedatives, tranquilizers, or drugs to control anxiety had about double the risk of hip fracture, and that risk increased to threefold among those taking larger amounts of those medications.

The message seems very clear. It is important to try to prevent osteoporosis; it is equally important to query older persons about the medications they are taking and to try to reduce the egregious overmedicating of senior citizens. There is very impressive evidence that overmedication can be harmful, one of the inadvertent adverse effects of certain medications apparently being an increase in frequency of falls and consequent fractures.

The average person over age sixty-five takes five to eight prescription drugs; some 400 million prescriptions are filled for senior citizens in the United States. There are several problems with all this medication taking:

1. Many of the drugs used are dangerous in one way or another for older persons. In 1985, an estimated 243,000 older Americans were hospitalized for adverse reactions to drugs.

2. A significant number of these drugs can produce mental depression, confusion, or agitation. It is estimated that more than 160,000 older persons experience severe mental problems caused by or worsened by drugs each year. That is of enormous concern. If any older person develops difficulty in thinking or memory, it is obligatory to consider the possibility that the mental functioning abnormalities are due to one or more of the medications that person is taking. This cannot be overemphasized. I know of older persons whose memory failed, who could not function, and underwent an extraordinary number of medical and psychiatric examinations at great expense before a doctor (or sometimes the spouse) suggested the possibility the suffering and defects were due to the multiple drugs the person was taking. In such persons, the improvement upon merely stopping the drugs is astounding. Unfortunately, it is often difficult for the doctor to get the patient to reveal the multiple drugs he or she is taking.

3. These medications may interact with each other to produce all sorts of undesirable effects—reduction in absorption of important drugs from the intestines into the bloodstream; reduction in absorption of vitamins; adverse effects on major organ systems, such as the kidneys. It is important to realize that there is an awful lot we don't know about drug interactions.

4. As noted above, some of the drugs can reduce mental function and increase the likelihood of falls and resulting fractures that in this age group can often be life-threatening.

Three case histories will suffice to illustrate these points:

Case 1: A sixty-eight-year-old woman developed modest anxiety with feelings of persecution. She was referred to a psychiatrist who prescribed a well-known tranquilizer. Her feelings of anxiety diminished, but she began acting strangely, was very lethargic, and complained of profound weakness. Soon her anxiety returned. Then she was examined by her general practitioner. He found no new abnormalities and noted that her blood pressure was normal at 115/70 and her heart rhythm, which had been giving her trouble, was quite normal. The psychiatrist, knowing her general physical examination was normal, increased the dosage of the tranquilizer. During the next two weeks, all her symptoms worsened. It was only then that her husband called the doctors and reminded them that his wife's usual blood pressure was 165/86. Only then did the doctors realize that the tranquilizer drug was reacting with the drug she took to keep her heart rhythm normal and producing a reduction in her blood pressure. The 115/70 was in the normal range, but in her case represented low blood pressure compared to her normal pressure. The heart medicine was stopped, her blood pressure returned to her normal level and her new symptoms disappeared, including the weakness and the recent anxiety that turned out to be a reaction to her feelings of terrible weakness.

Case 2: A sixty-year old man was found to have high blood pressure. He was given thiazide drugs to increase loss of fluids through the kidneys and thus lower his blood pressure. At first, his blood pressure elevation seemed to come under control, but then it got worse and he developed profound weakness that literally ruined his daily existence. This got progressively worse for months despite an increasing dosage of thiazides. In desperation, he went to another physician who took a careful history and found out that after the first doctor prescribed thiazides, a second physician prescribed an anti-inflammatory drug because of complaints of aching joints. The two drugs together are dangerous; the anti-inflammatory drug reduces the blood-pressure-lowering effects of the thiazides and together they can produce a striking lowering of sodium levels that can lead to profound weakness. In this case, the first doctor, not knowing about the anti-inflammatory drug, compounded the problem by increasing the dose of the thiazide; this resulted in a marked lowering of potassium levels, which in turn increased the weakness. Blood levels of sodium and potassium were found to be very low. Both drugs were stopped, the sodium and potassium levels returned to normal, the weakness disappeared, and then thiazides were again administered, this time without any other drugs, with subsequent control of the high blood pressure.

In this case, the drugs were purchased at different pharmacies and the doctor prescribing the thiazides to control the blood pressure was never told by the patient that he was taking a medication for his joint complaints.

Case 3: A seventy-two-year-old man suffered from clots in the legs for which he was given anticoagulant pills to prevent blood clotting. Studies of blood specimens showed inadequate effects of the medication on the blood, a somewhat surprising finding, so the dosage was increased substantially until the desired effect was reached. He was scheduled for weekly blood tests, but failed to keep one appointment and a week later died of bleeding into the head. Subsequent discussions with his wife then revealed the following: he recently had experienced trouble sleeping so he took barbiturates that he had obtained from another doctor almost a year ago. Two weeks before his death, he ran out of barbiturates and took no sleeping medication at all. Now the reasons for the avoidable death became clear. The barbiturates act on the liver and will increase the inactivation of the anticoagulant. As a result, the blood tests indicated more anticoagulant was needed and the dose was increased. The doctor unfortunately was not aware that his patient was taking barbiturates that were obtained from another physician a year previously and purchased at a different pharmacy. When the patient stopped the barbiturates, he continued the same dose of anticoagulant. In the absence of the barbiturate, the large anticoagulant dosage was not inactivated as much by the liver, there was an excessive anticlotting effect, and this resulted in bleeding into the head and death. The drug interaction killed this man. The doctor had actually asked about other drug use and had not been told about the sleeping pill usage because the patient did not wish to reveal the fact that he was using medications from an old prescription. A pharmacist might have warned of the drug interaction, but the old barbiturates and new anticoagulant prescriptions were purchased at different pharmacies. So the culprit in this case was not the doctor who correctly prescribed the anticoagulant, nor the pharmacist. Nor was it the other doctor who prescribed the barbiturate for sleep. It was the interaction of two drugs that caused this avoidable death.

This issue is extraordinarily important. It is estimated that one-half to three-quarters of medications given to older people are not needed. Interestingly, older people often get prescriptions from doctors and never have them filled or fill the prescriptions but never take the medicines.

I believe that every older person should be taking a vitamin supplement. Beyond that, doctors should be (but often are not) guided by the time-honored medical rule that numbers of medications should be kept to an appropriate minimum. Many of these drug interaction problems could be minimized if older persons taking more than one medication would purchase them at a single pharmacy, where the pharmacist could use a computer program that would warn of specific drug interactions. I should emphasize that adverse drug interactions or drug-induced chemical imbalances are by no means limited to older persons. They represent an increasing problem at all ages.

There are those who say there is no need for a woman to have a Pap smear after age sixty. I have never understood that recommendation, as about one-third of all cases of cervical cancer are detected after age sixty and one out of every four is diagnosed after age sixty-five; and 40 percent of the deaths from cervical cancer occur in women over sixty-five. Furthermore, in the past decade, a change has taken place in women's attitudes toward sexual activity in later life. To me, the data are very persuasive and the prudent recommendation is a Pap test every other year until age seventy-five.

Many experts would suggest a yearly prostate examination, but the evidence is flimsy. There are two potential reasons for doing the examination yearly—detection of substantial prostate enlargement and detection of cancer. If there is prostatic enlargement that could block urine flow, this will be detected in plenty of time by the prostatic examination done at the time of the left-sided colonoscopy that is performed every five years, or at the single interval rectal examination done between colonoscopic examinations. Besides, nothing would be done about prostatic enlargement unless there were symptoms (infection or urinary obstruction). The older you get, the more likely you are to develop prostatic cancer. Prostate examination is, at any age, an ineffective way to detect early prostatic cancer, and there is really no evidence that those whose cancer is detected by a routine digital prostatic examination have any different overall outcome compared with those whose cancer is detected because of specific symptoms. So the recommendation for those over age sixty is no different from that for those under age sixty.

Exercise may be important for older people in regard to osteoporosis prevention, but it is not yet established whether exercise after age sixty really makes a difference; and if it does, it is not known what kind of exercise is most beneficial or how much exercise is required. A study from the Honolulu

Heart Program published in June 1988 in the *American Journal of Public Health* found that moderately physically active or very active men over the age of sixty-five had considerable reduction in heart attack rates. That is very encouraging, but additional studies are needed prior to making any final judgment.

It is likely our immunization schedules will be modified in the coming years. At present, we give pneumococcal vaccine once at about age sixty or sixty-five, but we do not know whether it is really effective; and we give influenza and tetanus vaccines in the same manner given to younger people, even though we know the evidence indicates older persons often respond less well to vaccines. It may well be that older persons should get two doses of influenza vaccine or that tetanus immunization should be given every five years instead of every ten years, but in the absence of good data, we give all adults the same immunization schedules for most vaccines.

Although some studies do show inadequate response to vaccines, a very recent study by Dr. Peter Gross and his associates at Hackensack Hospital in New Jersey indicates that the response of older persons who had previously been immunized regularly with influenza vaccine was quite satisfactory. Whether this adequate response will be found in older persons with significant diseases or in older persons who have not been regularly immunized is not known. The importance of influenza vaccination for older persons is emphasized by the fact that 60 to 80 percent of all influenza deaths occur in persons over age sixty-five. A study by William Barker, M.D., and John P. Mullooly, published in the *Journal of the American Medical Association* of December 5, 1980, indicates that influenza vaccine was more than 70 percent effective in older persons.

If you are over age sixty-five and are a smoker, does quitting at that age or even at age seventy make a difference with regard to subsequent cancer or stroke occurrence? The answer for cancer is not known, but for coronary heart disease, the evidence now indicates that stopping smoking at any age reduces the risk of subsequent heart attacks.

A nutrition consultation is very important for older persons, and particularly for those with taste or smell impairments. Additionally, every person over age sixty should receive a one-a-day vitamin capsule or pill that contains folic acid. Older people may not absorb folates in the diet adequately and folate deficiency thus induced can produce anemia and neurological abnormalities. The importance of adequate folate intake cannot be overstated. A preliminary but intriguing report in the journal *Biologic Psychiatry,* in the spring of 1988, by Dr. Barbara R. Sommer and Dr. Owen M. Wolkowitz, suggests that with lower blood folate levels, older persons may not think as well as older persons with more satisfactory folate levels.

Studies are now in progress to see whether megadoses of certain vitamins can prevent some of the "normal" decrements in physical and mental function that accompany the aging process in many people. It will be years before such a judgment can be made. Until then, there is no justification for routine use of megadoses of vitamins in older persons. That won't stop the megadose acolytes and entrepreneurs, but the fact is that no megadose of any single vitamin or combination of vitamins has been shown to alter the duration of life, the quality of life, or the occurrence of illness in older persons.

If an older person suffers inordinate loneliness or depression, disabilities or inadequate support systems, a variety of approaches can be used, including referral to local centers, involvement in church groups, and so forth. It will take diligence, imagination, patience, and tenacity to help mitigate the problems induced by loneliness, inadequate support systems, marginal incomes, and moderate disabilities, but surely we must all make the effort. It is daunting to realize that by the year 2030 or 2040 there will be 50 million persons in the United States over age sixty-five, more than 1 million of them over age eighty, and that for many millions of persons, 30 to 40 percent of their entire adult lives will be spent in retirement. For too many the later years are, as Plato noted, "dreary solitude."

Older persons need the Health-Full-Life Program. It will not solve all their problems, but it does offer them the potential for improving both the quality and the duration of their lives.

There is an additional issue for older persons and that relates to sexual performance. As men reach middle age, there is often a decrement in frequency, strength, and duration of erection. For those in their forties, this is for the most part psychological, but by the fifties, there is likely to be a physical component, and by the age of sixty, most men are experiencing a significant drop in sexual performance—at least performance as defined by our society. That is particularly galling to men who mature well and acquire the trappings of intellectual, financial, or other success (such as acquisition of power) that make them particularly attractive to women. Vexed by knowing they are attractive but feeling betrayed by their bodies, concerned about what they feel are the sexual expectations of the women to whom they are attractive and attracted, they are susceptible to the lure of alcohol, performance-enhancing drugs, or any prescription or over-the-counter medication advertised as augmenting sexual performance. Women also undergo changes with aging, in particular, less vaginal lubrication; this can produce discomfort during intercourse and thus reduce sexual enjoyment. All this need not be so. If people at all ages would get used to touching more, it would lead naturally to a form of sexuality that can be every bit as pleasurable as intravaginal orgasm.

In the 1960s and 1970s, the "touch me" movements became very popular. Most of the groups were controlled by financial interests, manipulators, or power seekers, but they have left a useful, though often tarnished, legacy. Touching, stroking, and light massage are effective methods of very personal communication and at the same time can be erotically stimulating and a component of healthy sexual behavior. As men get older, they require more penile stimulation to achieve erection; if the couple focuses on fondling and touching, they will have pleasure and sooner or later this will lead to sustained erection followed by vaginal penetration. Besides, the prolonged touching and stroking create an intimacy that is likely to be very rewarding in itself. Both men and women should realize that reduction in frequency of insertive penile-vaginal sex is no big deal. All that is required in most cases, at least for men in their sixties and early seventies, is some patience and some extra stimulation, as well as a willingness to explore other avenues to sexual satisfaction.

That brings me to the sensitive issue of oral-genital sex. It is astounding how many people think this subject is taboo or that oral-genital sex is somehow "dirty."

The fact is that many men and women enjoy oral-genital sex more than any other form of sexual activity. According to a 1987 *Redbook* survey, about half the respondents, male and female, regularly give and receive oral sex. Many older persons, recognizing the desirability, as the potential for penile insertive vaginal sex decreases, of exploring other aspects of sexual pleasure, may either add oral-genital sex to touching and stroking or focus their sexual activities more frequently on oral-genital sex.

Are there any over-the-counter medications that augment sexuality or preserve sexual function (erection frequency, strength, duration) for persons who are middle-aged or older? The answer is no. The most interesting candidate drugs are vitamins, but there is thus far no proof.

Conversely, are there prescription or over-the-counter medications that interfere with sexual function? The answer is that there are many such drugs. I have listed some of the worst offenders in the accompanying table 12. So if you are taking medications and having trouble with sexual function, you should discuss with your doctor whether the medications you are taking can be causing the sexual dysfunction; if the answer is yes, changing to other medications or, if possible, just stopping the possibly responsible medication obviously makes sense.

TABLE 12

Drugs Causing Sexual Dysfunctions

Diuretics of the thiazide type (often given to increase urinary flow and fluid loss in persons with heart failure or high blood pressure)

Some antihypertension drugs

Some drugs for heart problems, such as Inderal

Cimetidine (given for ulcer-type pain)

Some antipsychosis agents

Sedatives

Antianxiety drugs

Alcohol

Methadone

Some antiacne agents

(The *Medical Letter* lists a total of seventy-five drugs that interfere with libido, erection, etc.)

And, of course, alcohol in older persons is terrible for sexual performance.

As regards sexual behavior for older persons, it probably is a good idea to try and stay in generally good shape. That means exercise and weight control. Flabbiness and a sedentary life are likely to lead to loss of energy and enthusiasm—and that is not good for sexual performance. It is also well to remember that stress and fatigue are very bad for sexual performance and that anxiety about sexual performance capabilities, especially for men, is very likely to interfere with that performance. So a positive attitude is very important.

3

The Exercise
Controversy

The exercise debate continues with no signs of a reconciling of the polar views. On a popular television show, a well-known cardiologist who has written a book on the myths of exercise debates one of the world's experts on aerobic exercise, who has written his own books and is an evangelist on the benefits of exercise. They accuse each other of misuse of data, come to no meeting of the minds, and surely leave the viewing public totally confused.

I should make it clear that I exercise a lot (I still enjoy playing squash tournaments despite decreasing proficiency). I favor exercise and I like it, but enjoying exercise is far different from advocating it as public health policy. It seems to me that assertions about exercise can be divided into three categories: documented benefits, possible benefits, and inadequately documented velleities—that is, hopes without substance. (I have summarized these three categories in table 13.) I should note that many epidemiologists would feel that some of the possible benefits are supported by such flimsy and tenuous data that they should be listed under "undocumented."

There is consensus that exercise can be very helpful, even essential, for many people in controlling weight. That in itself is a strong advertisement for exercise. In the Health-Full-Life Program, about half the participants seen thus far could benefit from at least some loss in weight.

If weight loss occurs with or without exercise, the cholesterol level often falls and the high-density protein level often

TABLE 13

Benefits of Exercise

Evidence Solid	Some Evidence Favoring but Far from Fully Documented	Undocumented at Present
Helps in weight loss	Improves bone strength	Improves the immune system
May result in moderate lowering of cholesterol	Prevents first heart attacks	Helps prevent depression
May result in mild increase in HDL	Prevents a second heart attack after one has occurred*	Is effective in treating mild to moderate hypertension
Makes some people feel better	Improves chances of survival after a heart attack	Prevents cancer
Makes some people think more clearly	Prolongs life	
May relieve tension	May help control blood pressure, and thus prevent hypertension in some people	

*In addition to direct effects, exercise may help prevent a second heart attack if it results in weight loss with consequent cholesterol and/or blood pressure lowering.

rises, resulting in a desirable change in these two major risk factors for coronary heart disease.

Can exercise lower the cholesterol in the absence of weight loss? The answer is not yet certain. An article in the August 16, 1985, issue of the *Journal of the American Medical Association* analyzed ninety-five studies and concluded that some cholesterol reduction will occur with exercise in the absence of weight loss, but the reduction in cholesterol was much more impressive if exercise was accompanied by weight loss. The same appears to be true of exercise-induced elevation in beneficial high-density lipoproteins. What remains unclear is how much exercise is needed to lower the cholesterol and raise HDL levels.

The other three benefits (feeling better, thinking more clearly, relieving tensions) are more subjective and involve enormous individual variation. It certainly is true that a lot of people feel much better if they exercise regularly. After exercise, many insist they sleep better. It also seems clear that for many people exercise is marvelously effective in relieving tensions; increasing numbers of people find swimming particularly useful in tension-reduction.

There is increasing evidence that exercise helps get calcium into bones and helps prevent osteoporosis, a disease responsible for most of the bone fractures in older persons, especially women. This supposition was based initially on the observation that rapid bone density loss accompanies forced inactivity; for example, a person who has a neck fracture and is immobile loses calcium from bones at an extraordinary rate. Unfortunately, there are just not enough studies using healthy adults to say with certainty that exercise will contribute significantly to both maintenance of bone density in later life and to reduction in the incidence of fractures.

Even if one assumes physical exercise is useful in creating stronger bones or reducing bone loss after menopause, it is not known how vigorous the exercise must be, how often it must be carried out each week, and at what age a regular exercise program should be initiated. The uncertainties are illustrated by a 1984 article on the effect of long-distance running on bone mineral content. Running did indeed increase bone mineral content, but among the twenty persons studied, increase was noted only for the "consistent" runners who averaged at least three miles a day; no such increase was found for those who ran an average of about one and one-half miles a day. But regular exercise (a minimum of three times a week), consisting of at least brisk walking of several miles or something equally or more vigorous, would make sense for every adult, particularly for women, in the hope it might indeed help prevent osteoporosis.

There are also increasing numbers of studies supporting the notion that physical exercise prevents heart attacks or makes recovery more likely after a heart attack has occurred. For example, Dr. William B. Kannel of the Framingham study, writing in the *Journal of the American Medical Association* of December 17, 1982, observed that the evidence did suggest that heart attacks in men—but not women—could be prevented by exercise. He also noted that exercise was less important than the other factors I have discussed, including cholesterol levels, blood pressure, and smoking. Dr. Kannel pointed out it was not clear whether the exercise needed to be vigorous or only mildly strenuous, and that there was a major difference between exercising and actually achieving fitness. Whether exercise in the absence of achieved fitness is beneficial is just not known.

The Centers for Disease Control published an overview in July 1987, when they reviewed forty-three studies on exercise and the prevention of heart disease. They concluded that the studies showed a reasonably strong protective effect of physical exercise and, in addition, that the amount of protection was related to the extent of the exercise; the more vigorous the physical activity, the greater the protection.

But according to other studies, the jury is still out on the prevention of heart attacks or coronary heart disease by exercise alone. If the exercise results in a significant and persisting fall in cholesterol level or rise in HDL, then almost certainly it will help in preventing coronary heart disease. But if you exercise and your weight does not decrease substantially or your cholesterol level does not decrease (or your HDL level increases appreciably), then it is very uncertain whether exercise will prevent heart attacks (or permit a greater chance of recovery if a heart attack occurs). Additionally, it is crucial to determine whether it is exercise per se or exercise-induced fitness that is important.

A very good article in the *New England Journal of Medicine* of November 24, 1988, highlights these issues. Men age thirty to sixty-nine were tested for fitness by an exercise treadmill test and divided into four groups of heart muscle fitness based on their ability to continue the vigorous exercise and on heart rate changes. Over the next eight years, those who were most fit were much less likely to die of coronary heart disease. The authors concluded that heart muscle fitness reduced the risk of fatal heart attacks. This article has been used as convincing evidence that exercise protects against heart attacks, but that is too glib. In point of fact, the article does indicate that exercise-related heart muscle fitness is beneficial in regard to coronary heart disease, but it also raises the question whether those who exercise are helping their hearts if the exercise is not vigorous enough to create fitness—specifically, heart muscle fitness.

Once a heart attack has occurred, can exercise play a major role in preventing a second heart attack? The evidence is somewhat hopeful, but murky and far from conclusive. The data were reviewed by Warren Browner, M.D., Deborah Grady, M.D., Stephen Hulley, M.D., and David Siegel, M.D., of the University of California in San Francisco in the August 1, 1988, issue of the *Annals of Internal Medicine*. They analyzed eight studies; in six of the eight studies, a 21 to 56 percent reduction in deaths due to another heart attack was found among those who exercised. The other two studies were negative. They noted statistical significance "when the data from these [six] studies are pooled." That summarizes rather well the status of exercise. You need to pool data to show convincing significance, and ignore the negative studies; it is hard to sort out the effect of exercise per se versus exercise's effect on weight and a resulting reduction in cholesterol and blood pressure; and for some people exercise after a heart attack can be dangerous.

It is also important to place exercise in proper perspective in relation to other risk factors for coronary heart disease. That exercise is of less importance than cholesterol, blood pressure, and smoking is strongly suggested by the fact that in Finland, among lumberjacks and farmers, the coronary heart disease rate has been the highest in the world. Many studies have shown that such groups smoked heavily, had high cholesterol levels and a great deal of hypertension, and also expended much energy in physical work. So it seems clear that exercise won't protect you if you ignore the three major risk factors. Now let us turn to less certain and more controversial areas.

The notion that exercise and fitness prolong life is attractive and comfortable. It would seem to make a lot of sense, especially to a sports- and fitness-oriented society such as ours. The study that has attracted most attention is that conducted by Dr. Ralph S. Paffenbarger and his associates. They analyzed some seventeen thousand male Harvard alumni who entered college between 1916 and 1950 through a questionnaire administered by mail. Then they carried out a follow-up questionnaire and analyzed the relationship between deaths that had occurred and heart disease, concluding that exercise reduced the likelihood of death as well as coronary heart disease. Their conclusion that exercise as an adult increases length of life by about two years has been greeted with great enthusiasm. I would urge caution; so would a lot of other physicians, including some of the most avid proponents of exercise. There are several reasons for caution.

First, about half the alumni sent the original questionnaire did not respond at all. Anytime half the people don't answer a questionnaire, you have to worry about biases and whether the results can be generalized to the entire population.

Second, some of those who were sedentary and lived less

long may have been sedentary at the time they answered the questionnaire because they were already sick.

Third, and to me of great concern, there was no measurement of either cholesterol levels or HDL levels. The protection noted might be due to differences in cholesterol or HDL levels, not exercise per se. That is a very important issue.

Fourth, the protection resulting from physical exercise seems to apply not only to heart disease, but also to other causes of death, including cancer. That, at present, makes no biologic sense.

Fifth, most of the reduction in likelihood of coronary heart disease applied to angina, or heart pain. The protection from an actual heart attack was marginal, and there was no protection from the most devastating aspect of coronary heart disease, sudden death. The most impressive protection was from "delayed" death after a heart attack, suggesting that prior regular physical exercise may aid in recovery from a heart attack once it has occurred. That possibility is supported by a recent study published by the Framingham program suggesting that the occurrence of heart attacks has not decreased but likelihood of recovery once a heart attack has occurred has improved considerably.

It is dangerous to advocate public health policy on the basis of a single questionnaire in which the self-reporting is inadequately confirmed by individual interviews and examinations. But the Harvard study does add some support for exercise as a protection against heart attacks, although we still don't know whether it is mild or vigorous exercise that is beneficial.

In the latest Harvard alumni study, most of the benefit found occurred in those who expended 500 to 2,000 kilocalories per week in mostly leisure activities; some additional benefit was found in those expending up to 3,500 kilocalories.

The issue of how much exercise is needed is increasingly the center of debate. The exercise proponents, some of them heavily involved financially, now insist all you need is a modest amount of physical exercise. The most recent Harvard alumni study supports that position. So does a report in the

November 6, 1987, *Journal of the American Medical Association,* showing that among 12,138 middle-aged men, the coronary heart disease rate over a seven-year period among those who did moderate leisure-time physical exercise was about two-thirds that of more sedentary men. The moderate-activity group expended about 1,500 kilocalories per day, mostly through lawn or garden work, walking, home repairs, dancing, swimming, fishing, hunting, and conditioning exercises. This and other studies will be used to try to convince the American people that only a little exercise is needed to decrease the risk of heart attacks. The evidence is not persuasive enough to make such a pronouncement. Indeed, although the *JAMA* report found lawn work, gardening, and dancing quite beneficial, the study on the Harvard alumni reported no benefit from such activities.

Thus, I can make no absolute recommendation. If physical exercise *is* beneficial, it may be that 1,000 kilocalories a week expended in physical exercise is significantly helpful—or 1,500 or 2,000 or 2,500. I do not think we know for sure.

Table 14 lists various exercises and the caloric expenditures for a 150-pound person; if you weigh 110 pounds, subtract about 60 calories from each figure.

If you believe that only 1,500 kilocalories a week is needed, then walking moderately fast for one hour a day would be sufficient; so would walking quickly for one hour three days a week plus vigorous gardening for two hours a week. I doubt that it is quite that simple. Of course, if you believe that 2,000 to 3,000 kilocalories must be expended, then you will exercise more vigorously.

It should be noted that if a person jogs at a pace of five miles an hour daily, that person will usually expend over 3,500 kilocalories a week. According to the latest article from Dr. Ralph S. Paffenbarger and his colleagues, that amount of exercise would actually increase the risk of death compared with somebody exercising a lot less. Of course, if you believe other reports, that much exercise is highly desirable.

If exercise does prevent heart attacks, it will be necessary to determine whether it is the exercise per se or exercise-

TABLE 14

Calories Expended by Exercise

Exercise	Kilocalorie Expenditure per Hour
Walking	120–150
Walking moderately fast	150–240
Standard ballroom dancing	240–300
Walking quickly	280–340
Vigorous gardening	300–360
Tennis (doubles)	300–360
Disco dancing	360–420
Jogging (five miles per hour)	480–600
Swimming	520–600
Running (six miles per hour)	600–660
Cycling (thirteen miles per hour)	600–660
More vigorous exercise	More than 600

induced changes in weight, cholesterol, and HDL. The evidence for exercise as a heart attack preventative clearly outweighs the evidence against exercise, but there are still a lot of unanswered questions.

Can exercise prevent high blood pressure or be useful in treating mild to moderate hypertension? If you are overweight, then exercise-induced weight loss may both help to prevent the occurrence of high blood pressure and be very useful in controlling mild to moderate hypertension. But we simply do not have enough information to predict how useful exercise may prove to be in preventing or controlling high blood pressure in a normal-weight person or in the absence of weight loss. The evidence on exercise preventing heart attacks applies primarily to middle-aged men, but there are recent reports indicating that exercise can reduce the risk of heart attack in women and also in persons over age sixty-five. Those are encouraging studies, but there just are not enough data to make any definitive statement.

We are all hearing more about exercise and the prevention of cancer, particularly bowel and breast cancer. Could physical activity actually help reduce the risk of certain cancers? The answer is that this is a real possibility, but at present the evidence is so fragmentary that no conclusions are warranted. It will probably take another decade before we will have enough data to come to even preliminary conclusions.

A study published in the *American Journal of Epidemiology* in December 1988, by Mary E. Farmer and her colleagues from the National Center for Health Statistics, suggested that exercise may help prevent depression. This is a very important issue, since depression is one of the most frequent illnesses plaguing our society. It would indeed be marvelous if exercise were effective in helping to prevent depression, but, as with the prevention of cancer, it will take a long time and a lot more studies before we have enough evidence to make a firm statement about the possible additional benefits of exercise.

Although I obviously favor exercise and have indicated that exercise may be beneficial, I want to emphasize that exercise cannot be called innocuous. There are many reports of heart attacks occurring during exercise, both in those who had been sedentary and in those who were considered fully trained.

Dr. Larry W. Gibbons, Dr. Kenneth Cooper, Betty M. Meyer, Ph.D., and Dr. R. Curtis Ellison reported in the October 17, 1980, *Journal of the American Medical Association* on two serious cardiac episodes among 2,935 adults, most of them under age forty. They concluded that "these data suggest a small but not negligible acute risk of cardiovascular events for adults participating in vigorous exercise who have been given a prior exercise tolerance test."

Dr. Paul D. Thompson and his colleagues studied thirteen persons who died during jogging or running and reported their results in the September 21, 1979, *Journal of the American Medical Association.* Some had experienced symptoms that could be attributed to preexisting heart disease, but others had nothing in their histories to suggest that heart disease was present and that exercise thus might be dangerous. Some had normal stress cardiograms. The author noted, "Exercise deaths do occur and there is no definite way to identify asymptomatic individuals at risk." The risk of dying during jogging is, according to a Rhode Island study, seven times greater than if sedentary; one death occurred every 400,000 jogging hours. Of course, it doesn't exactly help the cause of the avid, often uncritical, advocates of exercise that James Fixx, the guru of running, died of a heart attack at age fifty-two while jogging.

Although exercise may cause heart attacks or death, the risk is very small, and one could argue that those persons would have had heart attacks even if they had not been exercising vigorously.

But there is a new major concern that must be taken into account: silent myocardial ischemia, a spasm of heart vessels with resultant damage to the heart in a person who has arteriosclerosis of blood vessels supplying the heart. The spasm and adverse effects occur silently—without symptoms. They can be detected by exercise stress tests or monitoring the heart by a portable cardiogram strapped to the patient. Silent myocardial ischemia occurs frequently after a heart attack but, in addition, it affects 1 million to 2 million middle-aged and older people, mostly males who have never had a heart attack or heart attack symptoms. If a person has a significant amount of silent myocardial ischemia, exercise can make it worse and can produce significant heart damage. In this case, exercise can be dangerous. How can you detect these people before they start exercise programs and warn them? You probably *can* detect most of the people with silent myocardial ischemia, but testing is quite expensive—at present, hundreds of dollars—and the tests don't always uncover the condition.

It is my own belief that exercise is likely to be far less beneficial if you do not enjoy it. I see lots of joggers who look as if they were miserable, and I suspect they are jogging only because they are a bit hypochondriacal—afraid they will die if they do not exercise. Unfortunately, there are no adequate studies on health benefits relating to pleasure obtained in a given exercise. But it may well be that those who do not enjoy the exercise they have chosen do not benefit or may actually be harmed. Unless this variable is taken into account, glowing reports of the effects of exercise may be profoundly biased. Since for many claims, such as heart attack prevention, we do not have clear proof of the benefits of exercise, it makes sense to me to choose those activities you enjoy; exercise should not be equivalent to taking a bitter-tasting medicine.

If you do decide to start an exercise program, it should be done sensibly and, where appropriate, under proper supervision. A warm-up period is advisable, and if you have symptoms such as those listed in table 15, you should be checked by a physician.

In this chapter, I have been very cautious about the alleged benefits of exercise. I would like to end with a bit of a special endorsement for exercise. Preventive measures are increasingly being divided into those involving drug-taking and those not requiring such medications. If you want to avoid a heart attack, you must keep cholesterol levels as low as possible and high-density proteins (HDL) as high as possible. Blood pressure should be kept as close to 110–120/70 as possible. These days, you can take a drug to reduce cholesterol, another to raise HDL, perhaps something to lower blood pressure; or you can try to keep cholesterol low, HDL up, and blood pressure down by weight control. To me, weight control (including weight loss) makes more sense than taking numerous drugs that may have adverse side effects and undesirable interactions. For most people, weight control is made a lot easier by an exercise program, so if you need weight loss to control heart disease risk factors, exercise can be an invaluable alternate to taking medications.

TABLE 15

See your physician before starting your exercise program if you have:

Shortness of breath at rest.

What seems to be excessive shortness of breath after moderate exercise or inordinately heavy breathing persisting more than ten minutes after finishing your exercise program.

Chest pain on exercise—especially in the middle of the chest—of a pressing type, or pain radiating to the left shoulder or down the left arm.

Feelings of exhaustion out of line with the amount of exercise performed.

Irregular heartbeat that stays irregular even when taken while you are holding your breath.

Excessive pain in the legs after mild exercise.

A combination of persistent sweating and extreme weakness after moderate exercise.

Severe dizziness or confusion, fainting, a glassy stare, or a persistent cold sweat during or after exercise.

So there may be health benefits from physical activity, but we cannot make dogmatic statements about such benefits. For many of us who engage in a lot of physical activity, the pleasure of the exercise itself, the venting of taut emotions, the postexercise feeling of relaxation, and the help it provides in weight control are sufficient to continue our exercise activities; should it turn out there are specific additional health benefits, so much the better.

Is it justifiable to make a single summary statement about physical activity and protection from coronary heart disease and heart attacks? I have some qualms about doing so. Nevertheless, at present that statement would be that physical exercise, the equivalent of at least three periods a week of twenty to thirty minutes of moderately vigorous aerobic exercise at work or during leisure, probably does have a modest protective effect that adds to, but does not substitute for, control of the three major risk factors—cholesterol concentrations in the blood, blood pressure levels, and cigarette smoking.

4

Personality Type, Stress, and Social Supports

The Health-Full-Life Program has the *potential* for reducing the burden from heart disease, stroke, and cancer by perhaps 50 percent, but is that potential counteracted by certain personality characteristics, or by stress, or by lack of social supports? To many, the answer is unequivocally yes. That is part of the rationale for the burgeoning number of stress-reduction programs, most of which are variants on deep breathing, muscle relaxing, and thinking about either nothing at all or something pleasant. That may make you feel less tense, but does it improve your health or prevent specific diseases?

Let us look at the issue of personality type. When I developed the Stay Well Program in the mid- and late 1970s, Type A personality was in vogue. But in my 1982 book, *Stay Well,* I decided that the Type A personality was not a major risk factor for coronary heart disease. I said at the time:

> There is an additional factor that may well be of importance: the personality type. Dr. Ray Rosenman and his colleagues have for the past decade been interested in the relationship of personality make-up to coronary heart disease. Their group, the Western Collaborative Group, issued a major report in the *Journal of the American Medical Association* in 1975 suggesting that persons fitting into a category called Type A are much more likely to develop heart attacks. In general, the Type A

personality is epitomized by the successful American professional or businessman: hard-driving, aggressive, ambitious, work-oriented, success-oriented. The Type B personality, on the other hand, is more reflective, easy going, less ambitious, less consumed with the need for material success. Stephen J. Zyzanski, Ph.D., and C. David Jenkins, Ph.D., writing in the *Journal of Chronic Diseases* in 1970, summarized the characteristics of the Type A, coronary-prone individual: haste, impatience, restlessness, hyper-alertness, explosiveness of speech, tenseness of facial musculature and feelings of being under the pressure of time and challenge of responsibility. Persons with this pattern are usually deeply committed to their job or profession and often have achieved success in it.

How important is the Type A personality in the occurrence of coronary heart disease? Nobody knows for sure. If we accept the data from the Western Collaborative Study, personality type is perhaps the single most important variable. If we extrapolate from that study, the likelihood that a 49-year-old man with Type B personality would develop some evidence of coronary heart disease in the next twenty years would be about 140 chances in 1,000 or about 1 in 7. The individual with a Type A personality, on the other hand, during the same twenty-year span, would have about 1 chance in 3 of developing coronary heart disease. According to the study, the risk inherent in being a Type A personality remains highly significant even if all other risk factors such as cholesterol, hypertension, and cigarette smoking are removed.

However, it is entirely possible that there are subgroups within the Type A personality, some of whom are not susceptible to heart attacks. It might well be that those hard-driving, aggressive, ambitious individuals who are satisfied and happy in their work and who are successful are not prone to heart disease. In contrast, those who are hard-driving and ambitious but feel constantly frustrated may be more likely to experience coronary heart disease. In other words, within the Type A personality type there may be subgroups with different susceptibilities, depending on whether the individual is happy or unhappy, whether he/she has a feeling of self-worth and achievement or feels thwarted and constantly frustrated.

Indeed, in that very intriguing but little-discussed 1970 study by Zyzanski and Jenkins, it was found that there were three major components of the Type A personality—hard-driving, job involvement, impatience—and that these components were not correlated with each other. As they noted, it is not clear whether (1) the tendency to coronary heart disease is related to only one of these factors; (2) whether all three components are needed; or (3) whether one or two components plus something else is needed. The Type A personality is not then a single, monolithic entity; there are at least several patterns within Type A and the risks may be very different, depending on your pattern within Type A. Unfortunately, nobody knows very much about the Type A subtypes and which are more susceptible to coronary heart disease. It might be that some Type A subtypes are actually less susceptible. We certainly aren't yet ready to suggest that everybody with the Type A personality submit to psychological modification.

The Type A personality issue shows why it is so important to be cautious and to have a rigorous, tough-minded approach to medical recommendations. Since *Stay Well* was published, almost all the reports have questioned the Type A personality–coronary heart disease association. At the Society for Epidemiology Research meetings in Houston in June 1984, Dr. Suzanne Haynes, one of the most thoughtful investigators of the nexus between Type A and heart disease, reported one of these negative studies and offered four possible explanations for her findings, the last of which stated, "At present Type A is not an accepted risk factor."

I think that is where we stand now—Type A, long held to

be a major risk factor, is not, in actuality. The final prover-bial nail in the coffin comes from an unlikely source, the Western Collaborative Study, heretofore one of the concept's strongest devotees. They reported on a twenty-two-year in-vestigation of men admitted to the study free of heart disease in 1960–61, who were followed to determine the incidence of coronary heart disease and the risk factors associated with the occurrence of the heart disease. If the entire twenty-two-year-period was considered, Type A was not a risk factor for those who developed coronary heart disease.

Why, then, had this very reputable group gone wrong in espousing the importance of Type A? When the twenty-two years were divided into four periods, Type A was significant only in Period 1; the longer the study progressed, the less the evidence supported the importance of Type A. It turned out that if newly available and more sophisticated statistical techniques had been available and had been used in Period 1, Type A would never have looked so significant. That is quite a change—preeminent risk factor to no risk factor at all. It was also thought a Type A personality was important as a risk factor in recurrence once a heart attack had occurred. C. David Jenkins, Ph.D., Stephen J. Zyzanski, Ph.D., and Ray H. Rosenman, M.D., writing in the journal *Circulation* in Febru-ary 1976, reported that among middle-aged men who already had known coronary heart disease, the occurrence of a new heart attack could be best related to the Type A personality among the variables studied.

But another study, published March 21, 1985, in the *New England Journal of Medicine* by Robert B. Case, M.D., and his colleagues, found different results. They used a very sensi-tive technique called "angiography" that permits actual visu-alization of the coronary blood vessels of the heart and found no relationship between Type A behavior and survival after a heart attack.

All the negative studies would have buried a less resilient concept, but the notion that personality has an important role to play in heart attacks is very attractive and is not likely to disappear. Its followers began to suggest that maybe

Type A was not a risk factor but there may be subcomponents of Type A that were promoters of heart attacks.

A group from the Department of Psychiatry at Duke University Medical Center, led by Dr. Redford B. Williams, Jr., has been focusing on finding the most "toxic" components of the Type A personality and they, as well as others, believe they have evidence that the two critical features are the potential for hostility and the tendency to turn aggression inward. These results are based on analyses of the personality patterns of persons who have had enough heart problems for them to have undergone angiography, a procedure in which a dye is injected into the veins, permitting X rays to be taken of the blood vessels of the heart. That in turn allows the doctor to decide the extent of arteriosclerosis, the number of clots, how much narrowing there is in each of the three major blood vessels of the heart. The investigators then correlate personality characteristics with amount of disease of the blood vessels of the heart. There is an obvious problem to this type of analysis: to get into their study, you have to have enough symptoms suggesting heart disease to need an angiographic study. That means there is a very selected sample.

There is much uncertainty about the three studies analyzing patients who had undergone angiograms. All were positive, but in different ways. One study merely showed that those ranking high on hostility scores had more severe coronary blood vessel disease. A second study by the same group showed that the potential for hostility was related to the amount of coronary blood vessel disease but only if, simultaneously, the individual directed anger inward, so hostility alone was not the factor. The third study, conducted in Boston in collaboration with the Duke investigators, also showed that hostility and inwardly directed anger related to the severity of the coronary heart disease found on the angiographic study, but each was an independent risk factor.

Four other studies have been done in which groups of people have been analyzed for hostility and then followed for the occurrence of heart attacks. One of the four studies involved 255 physicians and showed that hostility was strongly related to subsequent heart attacks, severe heart pain, and heart attack deaths, but another study involving 478 physicians showed no such relationship. The third study, the Western Electric study, showed a direct relationship between hostility and likelihood of coronary heart disease and heart attack deaths during a ten- to twenty-year follow-up period. However, there is a major concern about that study; moderate hostility increased heart attack rates, but as the degree of hostility increased, the risk of heart attacks actually decreased. And a large study in Finland published in 1988 found that hostility was not a predictor of fatal heart attacks for healthy persons, but was only for those who already had coronary heart disease and high blood pressure. So hostility and inwardly directed anger *may* be risk factors for heart attacks, but it is not yet clear this is so, and if it should be found to be true, it is not known whether counseling to reduce the hostility and inwardly directed anger would actually reduce the risk. In any case, the Type A personality is not a risk factor.

What about stress? The literature on stress is so murky and conflicting that I will not burden you with either an overview or a selection of articles to document a particular point of view. If I did the latter, I could "prove" my point of view readily, but anyone trying to "prove" just the opposite could do so easily by selecting a different set of articles from equally reputable publications. One of the problems with attempting to link stress to disease is that there are multiple definitions of stress—external events such as job loss, internal stress as occurs in depression, or even specific physiologic or biochemical changes that are found in "stressful" situations.

Determining the role of stress, aside from different definitions and conflicting results, is difficult for many reasons. Certain stresses may be beneficial and possibly even reduce the risk of severity of certain diseases. That is, there may be good stress as well as bad stress. Individual reactions to an external stress may be profoundly different. A given event, say the death of a close relative, may shatter one person, but give another a sense of strength in coping with the bereavement. The assumption that a "stressful" event determined by an investigator is really stressful for a given individual may be erroneous. Some people clearly thrive on stress. Why should we then anticipate that stress would make them sick?

The following appear to be valid statements about stress:

1. In national surveys, a greater percentage of the public are concerned about stress than are concerned about cholesterol levels, vitamins, or exercise.
2. An estimated 150 million adults say they suffer from a significant stress episode every week. Over 50 million adults say they have a major episode of stress every one to three days.
3. It is clear that stress can make a lot of diseases worse, including hypertension, peptic ulcer, skin disorders, and heart pain (angina). Control of stress can be very helpful in cases of mild high blood pressure and in those with labile hypertension—that is, blood pressure that sometimes is in the normal range and sometimes, during the same day or even in the same hour, may rise into the abnormal range. Whether stress management will control more severe high blood pressure problems is unclear.
4. Stress can result in some very annoying symptoms, including: weakness, tiredness, insomnia, diarrhea, overeating, undereating, headache, back pain, and irritability.
5. Stress-related problems are thought to cost industry $150 billion a year in the United States.
6. Stress is considered one of the major causes of work-site and other accidents.
7. It may cause some people to turn to alcohol or illegal drugs, including heroin and cocaine, and it is one of the major reasons, perhaps *the* major reason, people take prescription and nonprescription drugs.
8. Stress causes an array of mental and emotional prob-

lems, including lack of concentration, sadness, depression, anxiety, and feelings of being "blue."

So there are many reasons for controlling and managing stress because of the stress itself and not because stress might cause a specific disease. Stress causes a lot of people a lot of pain; and that in itself makes stress management valuable.

There are a variety of approaches to stress management. Some individuals, groups, or companies that purport to help control your stress are irresponsible or even charlatans, attempting to exploit a national problem for their own financial profit. Others are very responsible. There is no one answer to stress. Some people need individual guidance, others find that group counseling and interaction are more effective. Among the most useful approaches is one or more of the following:

- Deep-breathing exercises;
- Relaxation exercises and meditation;
- Other relaxation techniques, including exercise and self-hypnosis;
- Learning to refute and reject irrational ideas;
- Learning not to turn every little problem into a catastrophe in a conscious attempt to put into perspective the daily stresses every one of us experiences, and to differentiate between a triviality and that which is truly important;
- Learning to substitute pleasant for unpleasant thoughts.

Sometimes an individual can, in essence, manage his or her own stress. But often the help of stress management experts is needed. Nobody should be afraid of acknowledging the presence of, or importance of, stress in his or her daily life —or the necessity to do something about it. After all, we are only on this planet once. A lot of the stress each of us is exposed to is unavoidable; and it is also true that many people thrive on stress. But for millions, stress becomes painful, makes life unpleasant, and can develop into the dominant feature of everyday living. If that stress can be managed and minimized, it makes sense to do so; for many people, reducing stress can markedly improve the quality of life.

So we are just beginning in our search to understand the influence of stress on heart disease and even on cancer. It is certainly too early to make any judgments or public health recommendations. The same is true of the closely related concept of social supports. Social support attempts to measure strengths within the society or family (is the patient married or divorced, widowed), and social isolation (number of friends, church attendance, participation in group activities). Obviously, this is a rough measurement; for example, an unpleasant marriage may not be a social support. Some of the studies are tantalizing: thirty-month mortality in an elderly population was inversely related to the strength of social supports; the stronger the supports, the lower the death rate. And it is well known that if nursing home residents are abruptly moved from one home to another, the death rate in the next year goes up precipitously; presumably, this is related to a disruption in their social support system.

In the renowned Alameda County, California, study in which 6,928 persons were followed for nine years to study variables that related to mortality, there appeared to be a reasonably strong relationship between social support systems and longevity. But the data are divergent. In California, social supports seemed to relate to the likelihood that Japanese who emigrated to California would develop coronary heart disease, but when Japanese who emigrated to Hawaii were studied, no such association was found. In Finland, men who had the least social support had the greatest risk of developing coronary heart disease, but no such relationship was found for women. In actuality, this disparity between men and women may be understandable. Women, during their adult years, are actually more independent in their daily activities, whereas men depend on their wives to fix their food, take care of the house, and so forth. When the usual support system is lost by, for example, death of the spouse, men may be much more vulnerable than women. As with stress, good social supports may help in the recovery after a disease (such as a heart attack) has occurred, but there are not nearly enough studies for us to analyze patterns accurately.

A recent report emphasizes the difficulties in interpreting the importance of social supports. Victor J. Schoenbach and colleagues from the Department of Epidemiology of the School of Public Health, University of North Carolina, examined social ties and mortality in Evans County, Georgia. There was a very modest relationship between the likelihood of death and social supports for white men, but the relationship was not very impressive and there was no significant relationship for white women, black men, or black women. The most interesting aspect of the study was the observation that social supports related to mortality primarily for persons over age sixty. I suspect that will be the major usefulness for the social support concept, and that we will focus more and more on attempting to buttress social support systems for older persons in an attempt to improve both the quality and duration of life. Supporting that assumption is a careful study of deaths in a group of five hundred elderly men in Malmö, Sweden, published in the *American Journal of Epidemiology*. It found that the risk of death about doubled among those with low social supports or among those living alone.

In summary, Type A personality is no longer a very meaningful concept, and we don't know nearly enough about the role of stress or social supports in producing or preventing disease. It could well be that in future years, we will put much more emphasis on stress and/or social supports, but that will be—if at all—for the future. Of course, it is important to have available stress-reduction programs for those who feel battered by pressures of external or internal stresses and for those whose moderate blood pressure elevation does not respond to weight control or salt restriction, but there is no justification for making stress reduction a centerpiece of a program such as Health-Full-Life. There is just not enough evidence to do so.

5

The AIDS
Epidemic

It is not possible to be infected by the AIDS virus and lead a healthful life. When people acquire the virus, some, perhaps most, will eventually progress to AIDS. Even if such a progression does not occur, to live with uncertainty is to live with a Sword of Damocles hanging over one's head. The constant fear that AIDS will develop is so depressing and anxiety-inducing that a healthful life, if not impossible, is at the very least very difficult.

In the history of life on our planet, there have been perhaps a half dozen mass extinctions during which large numbers of plant and animal species disappeared from the earth. In addition, man has been intermittently ravaged by massive epidemics that have swept whole continents and to a greater or lesser extent have changed the course of human history. Included among these are syphilis, plague, cholera, and influenza.

Plague ravaged the world for centuries, "depopulating towns, turning the country into a desert and making the habitations of men to become the haunts of wild beasts." In the sixteenth century alone, it killed some 100 million people in a world with well under 1 billion. In the eighteenth century, five massive epidemics of cholera rampaged over the world killing up to 50 percent of those afflicted. And in the early part of the twentieth century, one worldwide epidemic of influenza killed more than 20 million people.

Now we appear to be facing a new scourge—the acquired immunodeficiency syndrome, AIDS, caused by members of a newly discovered group of viruses, the retroviruses. Almost certainly this is a new disease that can be traced back no further than the 1960s. The argument favoring this dating of the epidemic is reasonably persuasive; the infections and tumors that complicate AIDS are so dramatic and unusual in their severity and complexity that it seems very unlikely the disease would have been overlooked. There is an interesting but at present undocumented hypothesis that the virus has been infecting man for a much longer period, but only became apparent in the 1970s and 1980s. That hypothesis rests in part on the fact that the sophisticated techniques needed to detect the virus has been available for less than a decade. If the AIDS virus had been around for a long time and infecting man quietly, there would have to be other factors present to cause such hideous disease now. One possibility is that infection with certain other viruses has increased recently and that AIDS expression occurs when one or more of these other viruses simultaneously infect a given individual. There is actually support for that concept.

But it seems more likely that this group of viruses has indeed been around for a long time but until recently did not cause infection. Recent mutations produced a variant that is now causing a ferocious disease, which is spreading at a distressing rate. As of the end of July 1989, there were more than ninety thousand AIDS cases in the United States and most of them can be expected to be dead by 1992. Of considerable concern is the discovery by French investigators of a second virus called HIV-2 that is quite distinct from the first discovered AIDS virus, HIV-1.

There are three categories of AIDS infection. The greatest number of people acquire the virus and carry it but have no symptoms and no evidence of illness. There are thought to be 1 million to 1.5 million Americans now in that category, although that is only a guess based on extrapolations from blood tests on small groups of persons. Some people think the estimate is overblown and that the actual number is between 500,000 and 800,000. Worldwide, there are probably 3 million to 5 million infected persons. There are three basic questions that these patients might ask:

1. *If you acquire the virus and have it in your blood, will it go away by itself after a period of months or years?* There are a few cases in which this appears to have occurred, but only a few. The general view is that once the virus is acquired, it will remain for the rest of your life, but, remember, we have only had a few years of experience. It may be another decade or two before that question can be answered.

2. *If you carry the virus, is there a point at which the virus will be inactivated enough by your body defenses so that you will not be a danger to others?* We do not have enough information, but there is no persuasive evidence that the body defenses effectively inactivate the virus. Once an individual is infected, it seems likely that that person can transmit the infection for many years, perhaps for that person's entire life.

3. *If you carry the AIDS virus but have no symptoms, what is the likelihood of developing symptoms or full-blown AIDS?* Here, again, we just don't have a definitive answer. Based on the available data, it would appear that each year about 5 percent of those carrying the virus will develop symptoms; in some groups, that figure is closer to 10 percent. The estimates about eventual progression to AIDS range from 30 percent to almost 100 percent. NOBODY KNOWS; we haven't had time to study the epidemic curve. It may be that progression toward AIDS is most marked in the first five to ten years and levels off thereafter; or it may be that there is no leveling off and eventually almost everybody acquiring the virus will develop AIDS. It does appear clear that many of those acquiring the virus carry the virus for many years without progression.

The second largest group are those who have acquired the virus and have some manifestations, but no evidence of full-blown AIDS. Persons in this category are designated as having ARC—AIDS-related complex. Manifestations include diarrhea, sweating, swelling of the lymph glands, low-grade fever, weight loss, and difficulty thinking. In some persons, the manifestations are mild and quite stable; in others, the symptoms are severe, and progression to full-blown AIDS occurs relatively rapidly.

If you have ARC, is eventual progression to AIDS inexorable and inevitable? No one knows. At present, the rate of progression from ARC to AIDS is about 10 percent per year, but that does not mean that after ten years all ARC cases will have AIDS. There just hasn't been enough time to make that judgment. Some persons with ARC have gone seven years and have been absolutely stable, functioning well, showing no progression. But it is clear that a large percentage of ARC patients will eventually develop AIDS and die. Fortunately, there is now some evidence that drug treatment can delay and perhaps even prevent progression.

The smallest number of people have full-blown AIDS, characterized by the occurrence of a variety of dangerous infections, several types of tumors, and often brain involvement. At least 80 percent of AIDS cases will die within two to three years, but 15 percent survive for at least five years. There may be a few patients who will survive AIDS, but the number will be very small in the absence of effective treatment. AIDS is still a death knell.

Nobody can predict the future with certainty, but two estimates that have gained general acceptance indicate the severity of the problem. The first is prediction by the U.S. Public Health Service that by 1991 there will be 270,000 cases of AIDS. The second is the estimate that the number of cases of AIDS, ARC, and carriers of the virus doubles every two years. If that is true and there is no change in the present pattern, in ten to twelve years there will be tens of millions of persons affected in the United States, and over 100 million persons affected worldwide. In central and eastern Africa, a geographic area with almost 400 million inhabitants, there will be, according to some experts, 50 million infected persons by the year 2000. Of course, that is only a guess, but almost everyone agrees there will be many millions of AIDS cases and that will be devastating for an already poverty-stricken and volatile part of the world.

It is an epidemic that may well be recorded by historians as the most destructive of the medical catastrophes in the history of man. Of course, predictions are fallible. The spread of the disease could lessen—or, alternatively, it could quicken. We may be able to intervene with drugs. The drugs that interfere with or kill the virus might change the progression from ARC to AIDS or might effectively treat AIDS and so reduce the death rate markedly. However, such antiviral agents will probably not stop the spread of the disease; to achieve that, an effective vaccine is needed. Because the virus is capable of rapid change in its makeup, an effective vaccine is thought to be five to ten years away, at best.

Homosexuals and bisexuals were the first to be affected in the United States. Next it was intravenous drug users who shared needles. Those groups still account for over 80 percent of the cases. Children born to women carrying the virus, and hemophiliacs who received blood products made from infected blood, or those who received contaminated transfusions prior to 1986 make up a small percentage. About 4 percent are heterosexuals who acquired the disease from sexual partners carrying the virus. In other areas of the world, such as Africa, the disease is centered in the heterosexual population among sexually promiscuous persons and their partners.

The question on everyone's mind is how to prevent AIDS. In general, the answers seem to be "safe sex" and education. Safe sex appears to have been defined by a variety of "experts" as follows:

1. Have mutually faithful relationships with a single partner whom you know well.
2. If you can't manage number 1, at least limit the number of sexual partners.
3. Do not have intercourse with anyone who has had multiple sexual partners (this is, of course, frequently not possible).
4. Avoid anal intercourse.

5. Avoid prostitutes; street prostitutes are far more likely to carry the virus than high-priced call girls.

6. Always use condoms or insist your partner use them if there is any risk of infection. Condoms, if used properly, do prevent transmission of the virus most of the time, but condoms fail to prevent conception about 10 percent of the time. The failure rate in preventing the spread of the AIDS virus is not known, but it is estimated condoms will fail in 10 to 17 percent of the cases. The use of a spermicidal jelly that kills the AIDS virus is also recommended.

7. Never have intercourse with a person who uses intravenous drugs or, for a woman, a bisexual man unless you know that person has had a blood test for AIDS and is negative.

Some would add two more components of safe sex. The first is abstinence for young people and those who are not married. That is surely safe sex; it is also largely impractical in our hedonistic society. The other is the warning that no sex is really safe sex, unless the partner has had a blood test and is negative. But even a negative blood test does not guarantee the individual is virus-free. Besides, I believe that is a mischievous suggestion and will discuss the issue more fully later in this chapter.

The following are the facts as we know them today about spread of the virus.

1. The AIDS virus can be transmitted by penile-vaginal sex. What about casual sexual contact with an infected person? The risk in a given episode of vaginal intercourse is well under 1 percent (probably about 1 in 1,000), but a single sexual contact with an infected person can on rare occasions transmit the disease; that risk is increased by multiple sexual contacts.

2. Anal intercourse is the sexual activity that carries the greatest risk. Several persuasive studies support the statement that both for male homosexual and for het-

erosexual intercourse, anal sex increases the risk about two- to threefold.

3. Despite what some people say, oral-genital sex is not very dangerous. There is an instance of a man who almost surely acquired the infection by performing cunnilingus (mouth to clitoris-vagina) repeatedly with a prostitute and another case of a lesbian-to-lesbian transmission, presumably by the oral-genital route, and there are several cases of homosexual men who acquired the virus but engaged only in oral-genital sex for periods of up to a year before showing evidence of infection. Even these cases among homosexuals do not prove transmission by the oral-genital route. These men were studied before a technique was available that might have shown the infection was acquired six months to a year earlier, when they were still practicing anal intercourse. The general feeling in the scientific community is that the virus can rarely be spread by oral-genital sex, although there is a tiny risk.

4. The virus can occasionally be found in saliva and tears, but there is only one case allegedly or possibly spread by kissing. Kissing, even so-called deep kissing, should not be considered a dangerous act.

5. The evidence suggests that an infected man can give the disease to an uninfected woman by sexual contact more readily than an infected woman can transmit the disease to an uninfected man by sexual contact. But spread can go both ways—man to woman and woman to man.

6. AIDS does not spread in households in the absence of sexual activity or sharing needles. You don't get AIDS by taking care of children with AIDS, living in the same household with AIDS virus carriers or AIDS patients. It is true there is one case of child-to-mother transmission, but this was extraordinary contact with blood, feces, etc. And there is one case of apparent child-to-child transmission, perhaps through a bite. Such cases are very rare.

7. You cannot get AIDS when you give blood.

8. Any needle stick can transmit the AIDS virus if that needle is contaminated with the blood of someone who carries the virus. So it is not only the sharing of needles by intravenous drug users. The disease can also be transmitted by acupuncture or tattoo needles that are improperly sterilized.
9. The risk to classmates of having a virus-positive child in school is virtually zero.
10. The risk to you of having a co-worker on the job who is infected with the AIDS virus is virtually zero.
11. You don't pick up AIDS from toilet seats, sharing combs with somebody with the virus, in restaurants or bars, or by being served food prepared by homosexual cooks or by homosexual waiters who carry the virus.
12. The risk of getting the AIDS virus from a transfusion is now less than 1 in 40,000. An occasional positive bottle of blood will slip through because of laboratory error or because a person may become infected and not show evidence of that infection on blood tests for many months. Fortunately, most infected people have positive blood tests within a few weeks. And the tests we have available get better and better, so the blood supply will become even safer in future years. Even now, the risk from blood transfusions is very small. However, that statement of reassurance does not apply to all areas of the world. In those areas of Africa where AIDS is rampant, the blood supply is *not* safe; a traveler to those areas who has an accident and requires blood transfusions is unfortunately at very considerable risk.

So casual, or even intensive, nonsexual contact is not a significant concern. Still, that statement has to be qualified a bit. Most of us are not in contact with the blood of others, and if we are, it is not direct contact. But health care workers are. There are a small number of cases of transmission of the virus from an infected patient to a health care worker who was inadvertently stuck with a needle that had been in contact with the patient's blood or had other very intensive contact with blood or body fluids and secretions. The current estimate is that following a deep needle stick or cut with a needle or instrument contaminated with blood of an AIDS victim the likelihood of transmission to the health care worker is about 1 in 250. That sounds pretty small, but to a surgeon who cuts himself all the time during surgery, it is scary.

In May 1987, the Centers for Disease Control announced that three health care workers contracted the disease by direct, intimate, intensive but transient exposure to the blood of infected patients. In these cases, the virus seems to have been transmitted through breaks in the skin or mucous membranes of the mouth. Such cases are very uncommon. However, any person handling bloody bandages of a person who is known to be, or suspected to be, a carrier of the AIDS virus or who comes into contact with blood (for example, a wound) should wear gloves. If the individual is not wearing gloves and blood gets on the skin, prompt, thorough washing with a disinfectant such as Betadyne is indicated. This risk is very small, but it is a risk and calls for common sense and good hygiene.

The frequency of infection varies markedly from one geographic area to another. In many areas of the United States, if an individual avoids sex with prostitutes, bisexuals, or intravenous drug abusers (or uses condoms for any contact with these three high-risk groups), the risk of acquiring the virus through heterosexual contact is minuscule. Even in an area in which there is a substantial amount of infection, the risk from casual heterosexual intercourse for a person who avoids prostitutes, bisexuals, or intravenous drug abusers is very small. What are those risks? All statements about specific risk are only reasonable guesses, based on several variables, the most important of which are the likelihood that a given partner might harbor the virus and the frequency of sexual contacts. If the sexual contact occurs in an area of the country in which there is not much AIDS, a reasonable figure for a single episode of sexual intercourse with a man whom a woman meets at a social gathering is perhaps 1 in 10 million.

If a woman has unprotected sexual intercourse for a year or two with a man whom she met at a social gathering and for whom she does not know the virus status, the risk increases to perhaps 1 in 20,000.

Suppose that same woman lived in a high-risk area such as New York City. The risk of meeting by chance a bisexual or some other man carrying the virus is much higher. But even there, the risk involved in a single sexual contact (assuming the man is not an intravenous drug user) is very small, perhaps 1 in 1 million. Even if she had sexual intercourse with that man for a year or two, the risk is no more than 1 in 1,000. So let's not go overboard about the risk of heterosexual activities. It is true that the figures will change as the virus spreads in the heterosexual community. But if one lives in a community with only a small frequency of the disease (as is true in most communities of the United States, in most colleges, etc.), and conscientiously tries to avoid the high-risk groups (bisexual men being the hardest to identify), then the risk from heterosexual intercourse is tiny and is similar to the dangers of being the victim of a violent crime, being killed in an automobile accident, and so forth. Even in high-risk areas, usually in some of our bigger cities, the risk is present but small for casual heterosexual activity.

Given the presence of a dangerous, infectious organism, societal reaction tends to move through the following stages: curiosity, knowledge, mild anxiety, apprehension, pervasive fear, panic.

In the presence of a rapidly moving, lethal epidemic such as plague or cholera in centuries past, progression from curiosity and knowledge to panic can be telescoped into a few days. This epidemic is moving much more slowly, yet in the last eighteen months, we have moved from curiosity through knowledge and mild anxiety to apprehension and in some geographic areas to pervasive fear. If public concern is not soon combined with public conviction that we are moving expeditiously, systematically, and intelligently to curb the epidemic, the inevitable consequence will be public panic. That may be hard to stop, even if we do manage to handle the epidemic intelligently.

There are already some ominous signs suggesting inappropriate behavior that could escalate to public panic:

- In Washington, D.C., the police used gaudy yellow gloves when dealing with a crowd protesting government policies on AIDS; they insisted it was to protect them from contracting the virus from somebody in the crowd.
- In Florida, a firefighter refused to transport a forty-year-old man with AIDS to a medical center; he was dismissed.
- In Arcadia, Florida, three brothers with hemophilia who were positive for the virus but showed no evidence of illness were kept out of school and eventually literally run out of town.
- In Michigan, a man who had the virus was charged with attempted murder for spitting on two police officers.
- The mayor of the City of New York suggested AIDS testing for tourists from foreign countries, a surprising suggestion since New York City is one of the AIDS capitals of the world.
- In one city, police were issued jumpsuits, gloves, and goggles to use in dealing with prisoners suspected of carrying the AIDS virus.
- Children carrying the virus are refused entry to schools. Adults found to be positive are forced out of their jobs.
- Men are accused in court of grievous assault for having sex when they knew they were virus-positive, even though the sexual partners showed no evidence of acquisition of the virus.
- In California, the male lover of a Hollywood male movie star who died of AIDS was awarded $21 million because the movie star did not tell him that he (the movie star) was infected with the virus. The jury ap-

parently was unimpressed with the obvious fact that the sex was voluntary and that the movie star's young lover offered no evidence to suggest he had become infected.

And on and on.

The seeds of public panic have been sowed. AIDS has been spread from child to uninfected mother (once), from mother to child through breast milk (a few times), from a man to his wife in the absence of sex (once), from a child to another child, probably by a bite (once), from woman to woman by lesbian activity (at least once). That means that on very rare occasions, it can spread in the absence of vaginal or anal intercourse—by kissing, biting, oral sex. There is no evidence at present that mosquitoes can spread the disease but eventually there will probably be one or two cases transmitted by mosquitoes.

If people concentrate on whether or not it can spread by kissing, biting, etc., and ask, "Could it occur?" the answer is yes. The risk is not zero, but it is infinitesimal.

We must persuade people to focus not on whether transmission of the virus could possibly occur, but rather on the extent of the risk. Whether the news media, lawyers, and some commercial interests will let us do that is uncertain. The alarmists and those who stand to gain may raise such a fuss about cases of rare transmission that public panic ensues.

If the pervasive fear or panic supervene, society will almost surely react with cruel, unpleasant, and draconian actions and measures, including many of the following:

- Massive job discrimination against virus-positive individuals.
- Increased anger and violence directed against high-risk groups such as homosexuals, drug abusers, and prostitutes.
- Attempts at quarantine of virus-positive individuals.

- Exclusion of virus-positive children from school and normal social activities.
- A barrage of legal actions against virus-positive persons for allegedly endangering others in one way or another.
- Denial of adequate medical care to those who become clinically ill from the disease.
- Severe jail sentences for those virus-positive persons found guilty of having sex with uninfected individuals (remember that in the not too distant past the courts in some jurisdictions meted out twenty- to fifty-year sentences to young people for possessing one to five marijuana cigarettes).
- Widespread obligatory testing for the AIDS virus regardless of the consequences.
- Great pressure on young people to conform—and not only in regard to the forms of sexual behavior deemed "proper."
- Pervasive discrimination and ostracism of persons believed to carry the virus even if there is no convincing evidence that individual is virus-positive.

In essence, we would be in danger of re-creating a modern equivalent of the Salem witch trials.

What about testing for the AIDS virus? Could widespread use of a blood test help identify those who are positive and abort the epidemic? No one knows. If widespread testing is done, there is, in the absence of treatment, no benefit for the person who is positive. They could be counseled to avoid infecting others by sexual activities or contact with their blood —but, practically, all they can do is await as best they can the likelihood of sickness. It is true that they can have regular studies of their immune system and be given certain drugs that *may* be helpful when their immune system deteriorates but before symptoms of illness appear.

There is an important difficulty with widespread testing that still has received inadequate public attention: the tests are not perfect. Some people will be called positive who do not carry the virus, yet the testing proponents treat that concern dismissively. They say that a positive result is confirmed by a very accurate test called the Western Blot, but in fact the Western Blot is still an inadequately standardized test. Results differ from laboratory to laboratory; what one laboratory calls a positive, another laboratory calls uncertain or negative. Add to that mislabeling of specimens and technical error and you have a serious potential problem.

Furthermore, tests, including the screening and the confirmatory ones, may be returned with the designation "indeterminate." To the laboratory and the doctor, that means not positive but not fully negative. To the person tested, it raises the fearsome possibility he or she is positive. And sometimes it doesn't help to "clarify" the situation by another set of tests. In one case reported in the *Journal of the American Medical Association* in the spring of 1988, a woman with no risk factors for AIDS was tested because the state of Illinois required the test for a marriage license. The tests were indeterminate three times in a row and devastated her psychologically.

If we start widespread testing, especially in low-risk areas, the majority of positives will probably be false positives. For those misidentified, the consequences will be appalling; we will see major depressions, panic attacks, and suicides. I know of a doctor who nicked his finger during surgery and was terrified that he might have contracted AIDS. He was tested, and when he was found "positive," became severely depressed, almost suicidal, only to find out that the test was a false positive.

It is hard to escape the conclusion that until we have tests that do not have any significant risk of false positives, we cannot opt for general testing—with AIDS, there should be virtually no misclassification. There are better tests now under development, but until these are available, we must insist that before anyone is labeled positive, that person's blood specimens must be tested by specially licensed laboratories on at least two separate occasions, and both specimens must be strongly positive. If there is any question at all, the confirmatory Western Blot test should be buttressed by a different type of confirmatory test. That is likely to be quite expensive (probably $200 to $400 per positive specimen), but the well-being of a great many potentially innocent, uninfected victims is at stake.

Then who should be tested? It seems to me that limited testing is necessary, and by limiting the number of tests, establishing acceptable standards, and exercising rigid quality control (all easier with smaller numbers of tests), we can pursue a sensible policy. In general, only high-risk groups who represent a source of direct spread into the heterosexual community should be tested. These are:

- All street prostitutes.
- Intravenous drug abusers who are incarcerated or enter rehabilitation programs (those who are arrested but not convicted should, the courts concurring, also be tested. All other intravenous drug abusers should be encouraged to seek voluntary testing).
- Much of the prison population, particularly those who are incarcerated for three months or longer.
- The military returning from areas where significant numbers of prostitutes are known to carry the virus.
- Those returning from stays of more than two months in endemic areas of Africa.
- Immigrants from high-risk areas.
- Pregnant women in high-risk areas of cities suffering from an AIDS epidemic (such as New York, San Francisco, and Newark).
- Those hospitalized for elective surgery. This would allow the orthopedists, neurosurgeons, and heart surgeons to know who carries the virus so they can take extra precautions to avoid contaminating themselves.

AIDS tests prior to marriage should be abandoned. When we have a virtually foolproof test and effective treatment, then everyone may benefit from testing, but concentrating on those about to be married is unwarranted and unproductive.

Most positive tests will be false positives, and that misidentification will wreak havoc.

If prostitutes are positive, we can do something to control their activities. Immigrants from high-risk areas who are positive can be excluded. Pregnant women can be alerted to the problem and be offered abortions, or their infants can be followed closely for evidence of infection. For some other groups listed above, all that can be done is counseling to avoid infection of others; in prisons, attempts can be made to have virus-positive male prisoners in cells only with other virus-positive prisoners (because homosexual behavior is a fact of life among male prisoners and anal sex is a major risk factor for acquisition of the virus).

Even then, testing of some groups I have listed could have undesirable consequences. Testing drug abusers entering rehabilitation programs could result in many drug abusers deciding not to seek treatment. Knowing that a patient undergoing an operation is virus-positive could make the surgeons so nervous that accidental surgical glove punctures could increase, or the operation could be performed suboptimally, or some persons needing an operation could be rejected for surgery altogether. And, inevitably, even with multiple tests, some defined as positive will be false positives and so will be mislabeled and mishandled. There are clearly some drawbacks to any obligatory testing program, no matter how carefully, cautiously, and humanely that program is carried out.

It should again be emphasized that our blood tests for AIDS virus exposure are getting progressively better, both tests for antibodies (that is, a body reaction to the virus that can be measured in blood specimens) and for antigens (components of the virus itself), but it will be many months and perhaps many years before we have tests that are so good that they can discriminate with virtually absolute confidence between those who are and those who are not infected.

Limited testing will not stop the epidemic, but it might slow it down. We should not assume that knowing who is positive in high-risk groups will result in desirable behavior by those tested. Of course, when a reasonably effective, nontoxic, anti-AIDS-virus drug becomes available, this will all change. Then widespread obligatory testing would be highly desirable because detection of AIDS virus carriers would benefit those individuals and would simultaneously help control the epidemic. Even then, a vaccine would be needed for full control of the epidemic.

The National Academy of Sciences says a billion dollars should be spent to educate the public about AIDS and AIDS prevention. Many educators and government officials talk of "educating" for safe sexual behavior in the third grade or even earlier. Far too little thought has been given to those who will teach the children, those who will teach the teachers, and, equally important, what they will teach and how the "education" will be evaluated.

We do not really know what sort of effect the "education" might have. There certainly could be some adverse consequences. For example, we are almost certainly going to use scare tactics. We will tell the public, in essence, that if they have sex they are likely to die. We are already telling them that when any person has intercourse with another person, they are also having intercourse with everyone that partner has slept with for the past five or ten years. To me, that is appalling miseducation. There is an extensive literature indicating that anxiety-inducing messages *can* be effective, but they can also be counterproductive. It depends on the content of the message, the credibility of the communicators, the socioeconomic status of the recipient, the level of anxiety of the recipient, and the psychological makeup of the recipient. Are we taking all of this into account? Of course not. We are developing kindergarten to twelfth-grade curricula that may be designed to inform, but in practice will be used to scare the students. Suppose we teach young people that expression of their sexuality is dangerous, but we offer them no other outlet for their restless energies. If we teach them that sex is bad or unhealthy or dangerous, will we see an increase in alcohol use, in use of marijuana, cocaine, and hallucinogens, in depression, violence, suicide? It is even possible that when young people are taught the potential dangers of vaginal sex and the relative safety of oral sex, we will have an extraordinary increase in casual oral sex. We are dealing with young, often fragile, ego systems. Miseducation can do a lot of harm.

We surely have a mandate to attempt to intervene in the epidemic by educational efforts. But lacking information about what will or will not work, we should investigate various types of messages; both negative and more positive messages should be tried with carefully conducted evaluation built in to each type of program—evaluation that will measure acquisition of knowledge, changes in behavior and attitudes, and possible adverse effects. The epidemic is of major magnitude, but it is not moving with such speed that we have no time to evaluate education programs. We can and must experiment with different kinds of approaches, evaluate them and use that evaluation to develop the most effective programs possible, those with the smallest danger of adverse outcome.

Our educational efforts must be age and geographic-area specific. It would be unwise to use the same educational program in areas in which the disease occurs infrequently and in areas of high disease frequency. In areas of low frequency, educational efforts might well be focused on avoidance of sexual activities with high-risk groups, whereas in areas in which the disease is epidemic, the behavioral goals would have to be more extensive. Programs in rural areas would be different from those in urban areas.

The age issue is equally important. We seem to feel that it is worthwhile to start educational efforts in kindergarten, but is it really necessary? And what will become of the children's perceptions of love? marriage? sex? the future? I would think it imprudent to start "education" about AIDS before the seventh grade. The potential for miseducating the very young is great, and we may do irreparable damage to their psyches and development. And we had better be impeccably honest. If we warn them against imprudent sex, we must tell them what the frequency of virus infection is in their area; if the risk is virtually zero, we must tell them that is the case.

What about education for high-risk groups, particularly

homosexuals and intravenous drug abusers? In the various studies carried out thus far, the general pattern among homosexual men following education and counseling is a reduction in the percentage who practice anal sex, a reduction in the number of partners, and an increase in regular condom use by those who continue anal sex. Unfortunately, a significant percentage still practice anal sex without condoms, and some do so even after being informed that they are infected with the AIDS virus.

The education results with intravenous drug abusers are so limited and so divergent that no summary statement can be made. In some areas, there appears to be less needle-sharing and more use of Clorox to disinfect needles and syringes. In other areas, educational efforts with intravenous drug abusers have been largely unsuccessful.

So education, like limited blood testing, is no panacea.

As I have indicated, you cannot lead a healthful life if you become infected with the AIDS virus. For the present, we cannot depend on antivirus drugs or a vaccine. It would also appear that those without AIDS virus infection cannot lead healthful lives if they develop an overwhelming fear of AIDS.

The following are simple guidelines for minimizing your chances of developing AIDS or succumbing to excessive fear of AIDS:

1. Remember that casual contact with persons carrying the virus is not dangerous. Besides, as the epidemic spreads, it will in many areas of the country be impossible to avoid casual contact with persons infected with the virus.
2. Recognize that the risk of transmission by kissing, tears, saliva, or even a bite is much less than the risk of being killed in an automobile accident or dying in an airplane crash.
3. Vaginal intercourse does carry some danger, even though the risk is very small. Most people are not going to check their partner's blood tests, but each person should be circumspect about his or her sexual partner,

especially in an area of the country with a significant amount of AIDS virus infection. Starting a sexual relationship with an individual who has been "sleeping around" in certain areas of the country is not a good idea. And having sex with a bisexual man is a bad idea for any woman. In addition, having sexual intercourse with a street prostitute or intravenous drug user is a bad idea unless you know the person's AIDS virus status *and* use a condom. In most cases, some careful thought about the partner and prudent behavior should minimize the risk.

4. Those who insist on anal intercourse had better be extraordinarily careful about the partner.

5. Persons who engage in fellatio and continue it through the male orgasm would probably be well-advised not to swallow the ejaculate if there is any reasonable possibility the partner might be infected.

6. Condoms are useful in preventing spread. Certainly, in many geographic areas with a significant amount of AIDS anyone engaging in casual sex with a partner whose sexual activities with other partners is not known should insist on condom use. I should stress that I do not believe that the well-publicized campaign for condom use will control the AIDS epidemic. There are too many people who just don't like condoms and will not use them despite concerns about AIDS.

7. When in doubt, sexual activities should be avoided or restricted to less risky sexual behaviors. Thomas More noted that "the race of delight is brief." If the consequence of one or ten or even one hundred brief orgasms is a life-threatening viral disease, then the price of those orgasms is too high. With a dollop of prudence and a modicum of common sense, you can experience the joys of sex and manage to avoid the scourge of AIDS.

In addition to individual actions, the larger society must take certain actions.

I would reemphasize that this epidemic is not like plague

or cholera. It is moving slowly enough so that we can react promptly but with common sense. We have to establish our priorities and then move diligently but systematically. Up to now, we have not been very successful with either task.

To me, the following makes sense:

1. We need a national antidiscrimination law with teeth in it. Those who carry the AIDS virus, but are not symptomatic or have minor symptoms, are not a risk to others, except through blood or sex. They must not be excluded from jobs, schools, or social activities. There must be no AIDS test as a requirement for obtaining a job. The Congress of the United States is considering this issue, but penalty provisions of the proposed legislation are inadequate to curtail discrimination. Until such a law is enacted and used as a model for similar state laws, widespread testing must be held in abeyance.

   There is a gargantuan problem about to complicate the issue of discrimination. Several articles in the medical and neurological literature in 1988 provide impressive evidence of early involvement of the brain in about 25 percent of persons acquiring the AIDS virus. Think of the implications! There are increasing numbers of cases in which thinking difficulties are a major *early* manifestation of AIDS virus infection. Would you want to be on an airplane with a pilot who was infected with the AIDS virus and might not think normally? If you are a businessman, would you want somebody with the AIDS virus operating your computer; if you are a bank president, would you want somebody with the AIDS virus and possible brain involvement giving financial advice?

   There is a likelihood that this possible early involvement of the brain will be used for subtle, massive, and very effective discrimination. Once the premise is accepted that *any* person with the AIDS virus may not think clearly, the potential exists for fervently denying any bias against AIDS victims while simultaneously practicing discrimination on the grounds of protecting somebody or something (passengers, children, customers, a business) from the inaccurate thinking of somebody with the AIDS virus.

The only way to avoid this type of discrimination is to insist on strong antidiscrimination laws. Nobody should suffer job discrimination merely for carrying the AIDS virus; the fact that the virus may go to the brain should be irrelevant until there is actual evidence the virus-positive individual has significant mental or thinking problems. It is a very tricky issue; and it also has legal ramifications. If a person infected with the AIDS virus commits a crime or after being aware of infection with the AIDS virus has sex with many persons without use of condoms, would not that person's lawyers claim diminished responsibility because the AIDS virus may have infected the brain?

2. To allay the fears of the health insurance industry and employers, the cost of taking care of ARC or AIDS cases should be borne by the federal government through a special yearly appropriation based on the cost of care of a given case (now $50,000 to $150,000) and the number of anticipated cases. That might be up to $5 billion the first year. Once that burden to health insurance carriers and employers is lifted, much of the perceived need to do prejob or preinsurance testing would be eliminated.

Life insurance carriers would still be in a difficult position. Solving their dilemma will require ingenuity. One possibility would be that life insurance applicants would be required to provide a blood specimen that would be stored. If they subsequently died of AIDS, the blood specimen could be unfrozen, tested for the AIDS virus, and if it were positive, the payment by the life insurance carrier could be limited to a specified amount (e.g., $50,000, no matter how big the policy), or the same payment limit could apply to anyone dying with a diagnosis of AIDS. Undoubtedly, there are many other ways of protecting the companies and still managing not to seriously affect premiums or permit routine testing as a precondition for obtaining life insurance.

Some people are calling for national health insurance to cope with the AIDS epidemic. I think that is a mistake. Let us not get bogged down in a debate on national health insurance. It makes much more sense to take specific actions to cope with AIDS rather than change our entire medical care system.

3. Once the antidiscrimination law is implemented, we must abandon anonymous testing for the virus. This is a society-threatening epidemic. To assess it properly, figure out which persons are likely to carry the virus without disease and who will progress to clinical symptoms, to monitor intensively for changes in the virus that may change the risks of progression, to keep track of those who need newer drugs as they become available, to intervene intelligently in the epidemic, we must treat AIDS like any other serious contagious disease. And that means the results of tests must be kept confidential, but the individual must be known to public health authorities. We have done this for many years very successfully with syphilis. Confidentiality is obligatory; anonymity is unacceptable for this or any other epidemic disease.

This is another very tricky area because with our intrusive computer technology, the question is whether confidentiality can be maintained. Clearly, it is not similar to confidentiality in past epidemics or previous decades. To protect confidentiality, the penalties for breaching it will have to be very meaningful.

4. As I have already stated, we should undertake limited mandatory testing. Prostitutes should be licensed not only in Nevada, but also in every state, and a monthly AIDS test should be required for anyone pursuing that profession, with severe penalties for anyone engaging in prostitution without the monthly blood test. I think it possible that AIDS can succeed where every society has failed and markedly reduce street prostitution, at least

in the United States. Many street prostitutes are now infected and many more will be before this epidemic is controlled. Presumably, the number of customers will dwindle as fear of acquiring the infection from prostitutes grows.

There are many other smaller issues that will arise that will have to be dealt with. For example:

- Suppose you drive by an accident, stop to help, and find that one or more persons are bleeding. You want to try to stop the bleeding, but you wonder about the possibility of AIDS. I think the best approach is to have a pair of rubber gloves in the car so you can put them on in an emergency. Emergency medical units instruct their personnel to use gloves in similar situations.
- Suppose a person is bitten by another person and the bite penetrates the skin. The wound should be encouraged to bleed and an iodine-like disinfectant applied immediately. In addition, I believe that the person doing the biting should be compelled to have an AIDS blood test; this will usually be negative. I think the bite victim is entitled to peace of mind. If the biter is virus-positive, the chances of transmission are very small; a blood test on the victim at one and six months would in almost all cases provide the needed assurance.
- Suppose a person is virus-positive and has a nosebleed while working. Actually, that person is not a risk to others unless they have direct contact with the blood, and even then the risk is minuscule. The person with the nosebleed should be instructed to place the handkerchiefs or other materials used to staunch the bleeding in a plastic bag and then disinfect them in Clorox.

There will be literally hundreds of similar situations; most can be dealt with rather easily.

There is another issue that must be addressed and that is

the emerging concern about the link between cocaine and AIDS.

The United States is in the throes of a horrendous cocaine epidemic. The drug can be taken nasally, by injection, or by smoking (crack). Crack, when smoked, causes dependency with astounding rapidity. New data indicate that cocaine use is associated quite strongly with acquisition of certain sexually transmitted diseases (such as gonorrhea, syphilis, chlamydia), probably because cocaine is a stimulant and cocaine-users are much more likely to engage in promiscuous, extensive, and unprotected sexual activities. It is also known that those sexually transmitted diseases are related to acquisition of the AIDS virus. First it was shown that those with genital ulcers in Africa were much more likely to acquire the AIDS virus during sexual activities. Now there are data suggesting that chlamydia infections predispose to acquiring the AIDS virus and also some very preliminary data in the United States suggesting that herpes virus infection may make it easier to acquire the AIDS virus during sexual intercourse.

The implications are mind-boggling. Intravenous drug abusers spread the AIDS virus by sharing needles. Intravenous cocaine users are at very great risk of acquiring the AIDS virus. Now we have in the United States the following dangerous scenario:

1. The cocaine-crack epidemic is out of hand.
2. Cocaine-crack use promotes increased sexual activity.
3. Increased promiscuous sexual activity among cocaine-crack users increases their infection rates of common sexually transmitted diseases.
4. Those who acquire these sexually transmitted diseases may then be more likely to acquire the AIDS virus during further sexual activity.

And, of course, there is no effective treatment for this virus; those who acquire it are likely to eventually die of it.

So you don't need intravenous use of cocaine to increase the risk of acquiring the AIDS virus; smoking crack or taking cocaine nasally may result in the same outcome by a less direct route.

Crack-cocaine may be the wedge for the AIDS virus to spread into the general heterosexual community. We are a pleasure-oriented society, addicted to violence on television and in the movies, and a society that places a great emphasis on physical sex. Cocaine is a stimulant that energizes, gives people a feeling of great power and potency, and encourages increased sexual activity. It is also a drug that promotes violent behavior. We cannot seem to control the supply and there is no known predictable and effective treatment for cocaine dependency. It will be very difficult to persuade young people in our schools to either avoid or stop cocaine use when the drug so relates to the violence that dominates our "amusement" industry and to the societal focus on the physical aspects of sex, which, as portrayed in the motion pictures, on television, and in magazines, emphasizes tawdry aspects of sexuality. Cocaine abuse unfortunately meshes with certain of our societal values. It is therefore very hard to control.

Since it promotes violence, promiscuous (not loving) sexuality, sexually transmitted diseases, and AIDS, and in view of the fact that it can do all these things even if taken nasally or as crack (smoked), we had better realize that we are now in the midst of an exploding epidemic that must be controlled; if we do not control it by reducing supply, education in the schools, severe punishment for major suppliers, significant penalties for users (including athletes, lawyers, doctors), and by well-funded efforts to make treatment more effective, then we are likely to face a national catastrophe.

As terrible as the AIDS epidemic is, some good will result from it:

- The medical advances from the intensive scientific attack on AIDS are even now extensive, and will be more so in the future. The scientific discoveries will help enormously in understanding the way the body functions. What we learn will make a major contribution to controlling both infectious diseases and cancer.

- The epidemic will restore choice to young people not ready to enter into sexual activities. The coercive peer group pressures so effective and destructive in the past will be irrevocably weakened when young persons reject involvement on the grounds of fear of AIDS. Those who desire sexual activities will continue to participate, albeit hopefully more prudently, but the growing number who do not wish such involvement will be free to make that decision without fear of some sort of peer group retribution or rejection.
- The AIDS epidemic may well result in a reduction in the ability of the drug subculture to recruit new intravenous users of cocaine and heroin because of fear of needle contamination; and it may convince established intravenous drug abusers to either stop using that method or to seek help. If recruitment of neophytes into the needle-using drug subculture is to be reduced, a vigorous, tough, and impeccably honest education program will be needed in every junior and senior high school in the United States.
- The educational focus on safe sex will dwell on sexual pleasures that do not necessarily include vaginal or anal intercourse. That public campaign will almost certainly influence sexually active people to focus more on the pleasures of erotic fondling and genital play rather than penile-vaginal intercourse. That, in turn, may actually enhance sexual enjoyment and demonstrate convincingly that there is a lot more to sex than perfunctory caressing, followed by rapid penetration, followed by a frequently brief period until orgasm.
- The epidemic may even place hedonism in perspective and thus reverse the dangerous drift of our materialistic society toward a dominance of sensate pleasure.

Eventually, we will have effective drugs and a vaccine, but surely the AIDS epidemic will get much worse in the next few years. It will challenge our common sense, our compassion, our humanity. If we fail to meet this challenge rationally and intelligently, the disease itself, abetted by our misguided actions, can threaten the very viability of our society.

6

Health-Full-Life
Nutrition

The Health-Full-Life Program focuses on five aspects of nutrition: weight loss to help control cholesterol and high-density protein levels, blood pressure, and high blood sugar; calcium intake; the amount of fiber in the diet; ingestion of cruciferous vegetables; and sufficient carotene.

Weight Control

If you want to lose weight, you have to reduce caloric intake. Most of the weight-loss diets are quick fixes in which there is rapid loss, often of body water only; but after stopping the diet, rapid weight gain occurs. Some of these quick-fix diets are dangerous, but there are some perfectly reasonable regimens that attempt the gradual, intelligent weight loss we endorse. The following are some sensible weight-control guidelines (see table 16 for summary):

1. Reduce total caloric intake. This means, in large part, willpower rather than fancy diets. Some type of daily record delineating food and caloric intake is virtually a must.
2. If you are accustomed to beer and other alcoholic drinks, you must cut your intake drastically.
3. Reduce fat intake.
4. Learn to read the ingredients of the packaged food you eat. The law requires a listing according to percentage of the product for any given ingredient. Look for the first two or three substances listed.

   For example, cottage cheese is thought to be very

TABLE 16

Weight Control Suggestions

1. Cut down on individual portions of main courses.

2. Cut down on beef and pork. Use only lean cuts or low-fat hamburger.

3. Eat very little of the following: frankfurters, bologna, bacon, sausage, salami.

4. Reduce by 50 percent your intake of butter and all cheeses (except skim-milk cottage cheese).

5. Eat more chicken, turkey, fish, and veal.

6. Make a meal of salads.

7. Eat fruits for dessert.

8. Reduce markedly your intake of whole milk, ice cream, soft ice cream; instead, use more low-calorie yogurt.

9. Increase your intake of cooked and uncooked vegetables.

10. Cut out between-meal and bedtime snacks. If you must snack, try yogurt or fruit.

---

good for those trying to reduce. Unfortunately, many cottage cheeses are made with whole milk and are full of saturated fats. On the other hand, cottage cheese made with skimmed milk is a valuable component of a reducing diet. Read the label.

5. Reduce the portions and the frequency of use of meats such as beef and pork. Beef, no matter how lean, contains 20 to 40 percent fat. Hamburgers, sausage, and frankfurters are filled with fat and calories; their use has to be markedly restricted.

6. Use more chicken and veal. These are low in calories, cholesterol, and saturated fats.

7. To some extent, overweight may well be in part a manifestation of salt and water retention. It thus makes sense to restrict sodium intake moderately, and cut down on the amount of salt added to food and the amount used in cooking.

8. In cooking foods, avoid the use of Crisco, which is saturated fat, and use corn oil or peanut oil. Corn oil is polyunsaturated and desirable; peanut oil is monounsaturated. Better yet, become accustomed to something such as Pam Cooking Spray, a vegetable-oil product that is completely free of cholesterol and sodium. Because it is sprayed onto the cooking surface, very little is needed for successful food preparation—a typical serving contains only seven calories.

9. Limit pies, cakes, pastry, nondiet soft drinks, and ice cream.

10. Increase the use of vegetables and fruits.

Obviously, you have to weigh yourself regularly and pay attention to what you eat. The following four-stage approach was suggested to me and seems to make a lot of sense:

Step 1. Weigh yourself on the same reasonably accurate scale at least three times a week, taking the average of three successive readings each time you weigh yourself. Follow the recommendations above and in the tables. Try to lose one to three pounds weekly.

If Step 1 doesn't work in one month, try:

Step 2. Graph your weight and try more willpower in regard to the recommendations. If you are exercising infrequently, increase the amount of exercise to a modest degree (with the usual precautions against overdoing it).

If this doesn't work in a few weeks:

Step 3. List all foods. If you still don't lose weight, use a calorie counter with a planned intake of no more than 1,200 calories a day for a woman and 1,600 calories a day for a man.

If all the above doesn't help within two to three months, you need *Step 4,* a structured program under the guidance of a good nutritionist.

Nobody should suggest that losing weight is easy. The world is full of culinary temptations. But reasonable weight loss can be achieved, and a program of regular exercise can be of inestimable value in weight control in conjunction with a sensible diet. Obviously, you can lose weight without exercise, but an exercise program frequently makes a major contribution to achieving weight goals and allows the individual to adopt a far less restrictive diet.

A sensible dietary regimen plus cautious exercise is far better than following the heavily advertised rapid weight loss programs or the guaranteed-to-be-effective fad diets used by so many people.

Calcium

Calcium is presumably important in the prevention of osteoporosis. It may also help control hypertension or even prevent it, and recent studies suggest that it may play a significant role in prevention of bowel cancer. But we don't really *know* whether calcium taken in the diet or as a supplement will be effective in preventing either high blood pressure or bowel cancer, and we cannot define its precise role in osteoporosis prevention.

The American diet is low in calcium, and the older recommendation of 800 milligrams of calcium a day is not adequate. Health-Full-Life recommends 1,000 milligrams a day for a man, 1,200 milligrams a day for a woman under age forty and 1,500 milligrams a day for a woman over forty. Intake above 2,000 milligrams a day is not advisable because excessive calcium can result in kidney stones. About 75 percent of our calcium intake is derived from dairy products. Milk, skimmed milk, yogurt, ice cream are all high in calcium, as are many cheeses. Green, leafy vegetables supply some, as does canned fish (salmon, sardines). Three glasses of skimmed milk provide about 900 milligrams. Cheeses vary markedly; particularly high in calcium are Parmesan, Gruyère, Romano, Swiss, Cheddar, Muenster, and mozzarella, whereas cottage cheese contains less. One slice of packaged Swiss cheese provides at least 100 milligrams. It is obviously important to read the labels on the cheese carefully to assess the calcium content. Tables 17 and 18 list the amounts of calcium in high-calcium foods for those on an unrestricted diet and those on a low-fat diet. For most people, careful attention to these lists and thoughtful selection of food items should allow each person to have an adequate calcium intake.

If calcium intake is not adequate, a calcium supplement can be given. There are several kinds of calcium supplements; calcium carbonate is the least expensive and provides good amounts of calcium. The major issue is how much of a given calcium supplement is actually absorbed. Until recently, there were virtually no reliable data on differential absorption of one calcium supplement as contrasted to another. There still are not enough studies, but a good analysis using a new technique was reported in the August 27, 1987, issue of the *New England Journal of Medicine* by Dr. Mudassir Sibtain Sheikh and his colleagues from Baylor University Medical Center in Dallas, Texas. They found that calcium carbonate, calcium gluconate, calcium citrate, calcium lactate, and calcium acetate were all absorbed about equally after a 500-milligram dose by mouth and that this absorption into the bloodstream was very similar to the amount of calcium absorbed after drinking an equivalent amount of calcium in milk. That is good news, but it is well to remember this was a small study (eight men, age twenty-five to thirty) using pure calcium compounds, as contrasted to many calcium supplements sold across the counter); so more data are needed. Until multiple convergent studies are available, it would seem to be better to get the calcium in the diet; only if this cannot be done should a calcium supplement be recommended.

Obviously, it is important not to take an excessive amount

TABLE 17

High-Calcium Foods

Dairy Products	Milligrams of Calcium (approximate)
Milk, whole (8 ounces)	291
skim (8 ounces)	302
buttermilk (8 ounces)	285
milkshake	360–480
Yogurt, plain, low-fat (8 ounces)	415
flavored, low-fat (vanilla, lemon) (8 ounces)	318
fruit-flavored, low-fat (blueberry, cherry) (8 ounces)	345
Ice cream (1/2 cup)	88
Ice milk, hardened (1/2 cup)	88
soft (1/2 cup)	137
Cheese, American pasteurized process (1 ounce)	174
American pasteurized cheese food (1 ounce)	163
cottage, 2 percent low-fat (1/2 cup)	77
cottage, whole-milk (1/2 cup)	68
Swiss (1 ounce)	272
Muenster (1 ounce)	203
mozzarella, part skim (1 ounce)	183
mozzarella, whole-milk (1 ounce)	147
Ricotta, whole-milk (1/2 cup)	250
Ricotta, part skim (1/2 cup)	335
Parmesan (2 tablespoons)	138
Sardines (canned in oil, 8 medium)	354

TABLE 18

Low-Fat, High-Calcium Foods

Low-Fat Milk and Dairy Products	Milligrams of Calcium (approximate)
Milk, low-fat, 2 percent (8 ounces)	297
low-fat, 1 percent (8 ounces)	300
low-fat, chocolate, 1–2 percent (8 ounces)	284
skim (8 ounces)	302
buttermilk (8 ounces)	285
Yogurt, plain, low-fat (8 ounces)	415
flavored, low-fat (vanilla, lemon) (8 ounces)	389
Ice milk, hardened (1/2 cup)	88
soft (1/2 cup)	137
Cheese, low-fat American pasteurized process cheese product (1 ounce)	88
reduced-calorie pasteurized process Gruyère cheese product (1 1/2 ounces)	160
cottage, low-fat, 1 percent (1 cup)	138
cottage, low-fat, 2 percent (1 cup)	155
mozzarella, part skim (1 ounce)	183
Feta (1 ounce)	140
Ricotta, part skim (1/2 cup)	335

Protein

Tofu (4 ounces) processed with calcium sulfate	154
Oysters, fresh, 6	162
Salmon, with bones, canned in water (3 ounces)	167
Sardines, with bones, canned in water (3 ounces)	372
Shrimp, canned (3 ounces)	99
Beans, dried, cooked (1 cup)	90

Fruits and Vegetables

Broccoli (1 cup raw)	178
(1 cup frozen)	94
Bok choy (1/2 cup)	79
Collards (1/2 cup raw)	74
(1/2 cup frozen)	179
Kale (1/2 cup raw)	47
(1/2 cup frozen)	90

of calcium in supplements. A substantial number of people have lactose intolerance and cannot tolerate milk products. Those people may need calcium supplements. However, lactose-deficient persons can tolerate yogurt; before calcium supplements are used, a diet rich in yogurt should be attempted. Three standard helpings of yogurt a day should suffice.

Fiber

Fiber is the bulk or roughage component of our diets—those indigestible elements that pass through the stomach and intestines without being absorbed. Most fiber is from plant sources—fruits, vegetables, and grains. There are five kinds of fiber: cellulose, hemicellulose, lignins, pectins, and gums—all except lignins are complex carbohydrates. It is important to realize that different foods contain different kinds of fiber. If you listen to the fiber acolytes, they will tell you that each type of fiber has a proven benefit; supposedly, about thirty human diseases or disorders—including heart disease, high blood pressure, obesity, appendicitis, diverticulitis, hemorrhoids, bowel cancer—can be helped or prevented by eating adequate amounts of fiber. Does a high-fiber diet really prevent bowel cancer? The answer is that we still do not know. But it may, and these fruits and vegetables often have other desirable aspects, such as high-vitamin, high-beta-carotene, low-fat content.

We are also not sure how much fiber should be ingested each day. More is *not* necessarily better. Some sources, including the National Cancer Institute, recommend 20 to 35 grams a day. Over 30 grams a day is a lot of fiber. An article in one of our leading newspapers in July 1986 suggested 45 grams a day. To include 45 grams a day in your diet would be very difficult and perhaps dangerous, as too much cereal fiber reduces the absorption of essential minerals such as zinc, calcium, and magnesium. Some experimental studies suggest that too much of certain fibers can even promote bowel cancer.

In the United States, the prevailing philosophy is "If a

moderate amount is good, more is better." That is not always so. In an article in the January 1988 *Archives of Surgery,* Dr. James McClusken and Dr. Ned Carp reported the case of a man who ate two large bowls of bran cereal (probably well over 20 grams of fiber, the entire daily recommended amount) and eighteen hours later developed an obstruction of his small intestines—it was a ball of bran cereal that required a major operation to remove. Such cases, fortunately rare, have been described since 1932.

"Moderation" is the operative word. A diet with ample amounts of fiber is likely to be good for your digestive tract, could well be helpful to your heart, and might prevent bowel cancers. However, there are no guarantees. A minimum of 20 grams a day makes sense, but over 30 to 35 grams a day is neither necessary nor desirable.

Will oat bran, which provides soluble fiber, lower the cholesterol level? Two studies by a group at Northwestern University are quite hopeful. They added two ounces of oat bran or oatmeal to a low-fat, low-cholesterol diet and found that over an eight-week period, those who ate the oatmeal had a modest lowering of cholesterol compared with those on a low-fat, low-cholesterol diet only. Two ounces is not very much; one-half cup of cereal provides one ounce and the other ounce can be readily obtained by eating oat bran muffins, cookies, etc. It is well to note that the volunteers in these studies started with relatively low blood levels of cholesterol, and that most of the cholesterol drop they experienced during the study period resulted from the low-fat, low-cholesterol diet. There was only a modest further cholesterol-lowering when oat fiber was added in the form of cereal, muffins, etc. The total study period was sixteen weeks. Whether the results of these studies can be applied to people with higher cholesterol levels who are not on an effective low-cholesterol, low-fat diet is not at all certain.

Tables 19, 20, and 21 list the high-fiber foods and cereals, including those providing soluble fiber; by following those lists, it is easy to adjust your diet to get the 20 grams a day. For example, a medium bowl of high-fiber cereal, a few slices

TABLE 19

Foods High in Dietary Fiber and Roughage

Food Source	Amount	Total Grams of Fiber
100% bran cereals	3/4 cup	12–15
Wheat bran	1/2 cup	12
Kidney beans	1 can, cooked	12
Whole wheat flour	1/2 cup	7.6
Sweet corn	1 ear	6.6
Grape-nuts	3/4 cup	5.9
Pinto beans	1/2 cup, cooked	5.6
Broccoli	3/4 cup	5.0
Potato	1 medium	4.8
Pear, with peel	1 medium	4.7
Sweet corn, canned	1/2 cup	4.7
Baked beans	1/3 cup	4.6
Rolled oats	1/2 cup, cooked	4.5
Blackberries	1/2 cup	4.5
Shredded wheat	2 biscuits	4.4
Strawberries	10 large	3.8
Brussels sprouts	3/4 cup	3.4
Peas	1/2 cup	3.0
Carrots, boiled	1/2 cup	2.8
Whole wheat bread	1 slice	2.8
Brazil nuts	1/4 cup	2.7
Peanuts	1 ounce	2.5
Apple, with peel	1 small	2.4
Peach	1 medium	2.3
Cabbage	1/2 cup, cooked	2.0

of whole wheat or fiber-enriched white bread, two portions of fiber-containing vegetables, and two portions of fiber-containing fruit daily will provide the recommended amount.

TABLE 20

Cereals High in Fiber
(values are approximate)

Cereal	Size of Portion	Fiber Content (grams)
All-Bran with Extra Fiber (Kellogg's)	1 ounce (1/2 cup)	14
Fiber One (General Mills)	1 ounce (1/2 cup)	13
All-Bran (Kellogg's)	1 ounce (1/2 cup)	10
100% Bran (Nabisco)	1 ounce (1/2 cup)	10
Mueslix Bran Cereal (Kellogg's)	1.45 ounces (1/2 cup)	6
Nutrific Oatmeal Flakes (Kellogg's)	1 ounce (1 cup)	6
Crunchy Bran (Quaker)	1 ounce	5.1
Bran Flakes (Post)	1 ounce (2/3 cup)	5
Bran Flakes (Kellogg's)	1 ounce (2/3 cup)	5
Raisin Bran (Kellogg's)	1 ounce (3/4 cup)	5
Fruit & Fibre (Post)	1 ounce (1/2 cup)	5
Total Raisin Bran (General Mills)	1.5 ounces	5
Cracklin' Oat Bran (Kellogg's)	1 ounce (1/2 cup)	5
Raisin Bran (Post)	1 ounce (1/2 cup)	4
Shredded Wheat & Bran (Nabisco)	1 ounce (2/3 cup)	4

NOTE: To get a given amount of fiber, portion sizes differ. Many cereals have fiber content per portion that range from 0.5–2.0 grams.

TABLE 21

Foods Providing the Most Soluble Fiber

Food	Amount	Grams of Soluble Fiber
Black-eyed peas	1/3 cup	3.7
Chili with beans	1 cup	2.3
Kidney beans	1/3 cup	1.7
Oatmeal	3/4 cup cooked	1.4
Oat bran	1/2 cup	1.0
All bran	1/3 cup	1.6
Corn	1/2 cup frozen or 1 ear corn on cob	1.6
Brussels sprouts	1/2 cup	1.4
Baked potato with skin	1	1.3
Apricots	4	1.4
Zucchini	1/2 cup	1.3
Carrots	1/2 cup cooked	1.2

If you've been told you need more fiber in your diet, there are some tasty possibilities. Have you ever thought of . . .

- Eating potatoes with the peels on?
- Eating fresh, unpeeled fruit instead of drinking juice?
- Topping ice cream with bananas, strawberries, or peanuts?
- Filling your tostados, tacos, and enchiladas with beans instead of beef?
- Adding barley or beans to your vegetable soup?
- Munching on popcorn or corn chips instead of potato chips?
- Replacing low-fiber cakes with fruit and nut breads?
- Having a corn or bran muffin for breakfast instead of

Danish or some other kind of sugary, nonnutritional cake?
- Having oatmeal raisin cookies or coconut macaroons instead of sugar or butter cookies?
- Making your own breakfast granola with rolled oats, bran, raisins, slivered almonds, or walnuts and dried fruit?
- Topping yogurt with bran, sunflower seeds, or chopped apples?
- Leaving peels on apples when you bake them or turn them into applesauce?
- Rolling chicken in corn or oat bran instead of breadcrumbs for oven baking?
- Substituting whole wheat flour for white in your recipes for baked products (the proportions are the same)? Or the product may be made of half white flour and half wheat flour.

Cruciferous Vegetables

The concept that certain vegetables protect against intestinal cancer has been given considerable recent impetus by Saxon Graham and his colleagues at Roswell Memorial Institute in Buffalo, New York. Their study, which compared the diet in bowel cancer patients and in control subjects without cancer, found no differences in any aspect of diet—including meat—other than vegetable consumption. The bowel cancer patients consumed less cabbage, Brussels sprouts, and broccoli. These data are consistent with careful experimental studies by Lee W. Wattenberg of the University of Minnesota Medical School, showing that these vegetables contain substances that augment the body's defenses against certain tumor-causing agents. They are the cruciferous or "gassy" vegetables, and include broccoli, cabbage (or cole slaw), Brussels sprouts, and cauliflower.

In addition, there are experimental data suggesting that substances in cruciferous vegetables might decrease the incidence and/or progression of cancers other than bowel cancer; this would include cancers of the stomach and breast.

In 1983 and 1984, the National Cancer Institute, the National Academy of Sciences, and the American Cancer Society recommended dietary changes to reduce the risk of cancer; included in the recommendations was an increase in cruciferous vegetables. It is important to emphasize that there is no proof cruciferous vegetables actually prevent any cancer; some studies support those of Dr. Graham, others do not. Even if they do help prevent certain cancers, we do not know the effects of storage and cooking or whether vegetables from different geographic areas or grown at different times of the year might have different protection capabilities. But there is no evidence that eating more cruciferous vegetables will harm you, and as they might be beneficial, it makes sense to include them in your diet. However, there are no guarantees that cruciferous vegetables will protect against anything. So if having more intestinal gas shatters your psyche, you probably will not want to increase your intake of crucifers.

Despite some reservations, Health-Full-Life recommends that each person include a portion of cruciferous vegetables in the diet at least three to four times a week. The crucifers also provide other dietary benefits in regard to fiber, carotenes, and weight control. Broccoli, for example, is terrific for dietary fiber, carotenes, crucifers, and calcium.

Carotenes

Carotenes are constituents of certain vegetables and fruits. After absorption in the intestines, some of the carotenes are carried to the liver and transformed into vitamin A; the rest of the absorbed carotenes are distributed to most body tissues. There, they are virtually nontoxic and appear to contain impressive antitumor properties. Carotenes include several subgroups; it is the beta-carotene that appears to offer the most health benefits. Approximately twenty studies have come out up to now, most of which show that the greater the carotene intake and the higher the beta-carotene blood concentration, the lower the incidence of certain cancers, particularly lung cancer. Are the data conclusive? Absolutely not.

A careful study is well under way in Boston involving thousands of middle-aged doctors who are taking extra doses of carotenes daily; they will be compared with doctors not taking carotenes with regard to cancer occurrence over a period of eight years. That study should give some helpful results by the late 1980s or early 1990s. Until this and five similar studies now being conducted are completed, no definitive statement can be made about carotene administration and cancer prevention. But the evidence is now encouraging enough to advise that each person consume adequate carotenes in the diet. Carrots are the best source. Fortunately, cooking carrots does not result in carotene loss, so you may eat them any way that appeals to you. If you don't like carrots, other vegetables and fruits contain ample amounts of carotenes (see table 22). The recommendation is to eat one portion of carrots three to four times a week and one portion of vegetables of the dark green or yellow groups or certain yellow fruits at least three to four times a week.

One of the numerous studies showing protection from lung cancer by carotenes was published in the *American Journal of Epidemiology* in March 1987. The investigation, by Tim E. Byers, Saxon Graham, and their colleagues at the State University of New York in Buffalo, had several flaws, but nevertheless did show modest protection for diets containing larger amounts of carotenes. For smokers, the ones primarily at risk for lung cancer, a higher carotene intake may reduce the risk somewhat, but will do no more than that. The encouraging bit of information from the study was that the difference between the higher risk (lower carotene intake) and the lower risk (higher carotene intake) groups was the equivalent of one carrot a day.

TABLE 22

Foods High in Carotenes

Vegetables	Usual Amount
Beet greens, cooked	1/2 cup
Broccoli	1/2 cup
Carrots	1/2 cup
Carrot juice	4 ounces
Chard, cooked	1/2 cup
Chicory, cooked	1/2 cup
Collard greens, cooked	1/2 cup
Kale, cooked	1/2 cup
Mixed vegetables	1/2 cup
Mustard greens, cooked	1/2 cup
Parsley, fresh	1/2 cup
Pumpkin	1/2 cup
Spinach, cooked	1/2 cup
Sweet potatoes	1 small potato
Tomato juice	12 ounces
Watercress	1/2 cup
Winter squash	1/2 cup

Fruit	
Apricots, canned	6 halves
Apricots, dried	6 halves
Apricots, fresh	3 medium
Cantaloupe	1/4 melon
Mango	1/2 medium
Nectarine	1 medium
Papayas	1/2 cup
Persimmon	1 medium
Watermelon	4-by-8 inch wedge

Health-Full-Life Recipes

The following are a group of recipes culled from various sources—recipes containing foods that are *good* for you. There are, of course, many approaches to healthful recipes, and the ones we have included are illustrative of the kinds of recipes you should be looking for or creating yourself. For each of the recipes, we tell you why we included it, caloric content, and an idea of how much it costs. Since there are marked seasonal and geographic differences in cost of various ingredients, only three categories are used: expensive, moderate, and inexpensive. It is difficult to give exact calorie counts, and so, in some cases, we have had to make some arbitrary judgments.

Caloric Content

	Low	Medium	High
Soups and appetizers	Less than 90	90–200	More than 200
Entrées (main courses)	Less than 250	251–500	More than 500
Vegetable dishes	Less than 80	81–199	More than 200
Salads	Less than 90	90–200	More than 200
Desserts	Less than 125	126–300	More than 300
Breads	Less than 70	71–169	More than 170

Preparation will be divided into easy, moderately difficult, and difficult.

Salmon Spread

Appetizer/snack

*1 15½-ounce can salmon, drained (do not
  remove bones)*
*4 ounces firm tofu, drained well and
  pressed dry with paper towels*
1 small onion, finely chopped
Juice of 1 lemon
*1 tablespoon fresh, chopped dill, or 1
  teaspoon dried dill*
1 teaspoon white horseradish
1 teaspoon Worcestershire sauce
*Salt and freshly ground black pepper to
  taste*
Chopped parsley

Combine ingredients in food processor, blender, or by hand.
Chill until ready to serve. Garnish with parsley. Serve with
party-size pumpernickel or other whole grain bread. Serve
on romaine lettuce leaves.

Serves 8.

Cost:	Inexpensive.
Calories:	93 per serving (medium).
Preparation:	Easy.
Comments:	Good served with hot pumpernickel rolls or bread and surrounded with marinated vegetables. High in calcium; the pumpernickel adds fiber.

Curried Yogurt Dip
Appetizer/snack

4 ounces Major Grey mango chutney
1 tablespoon curry powder
1 pint plain low-fat yogurt

Put chutney into food processor and puree. Add curry powder and blend. Empty mixture into bowl and fold in yogurt. Thoroughly blend, but do not overmix or it will become watery. Recipe may be doubled.

Serve with platter of fresh, uncooked vegetables such as zucchini, cherry tomatoes, broccoli, cauliflower, cucumber, carrots, celery, radishes.

Serves 8 to 10.

Cost:	Inexpensive to moderate.
Calories:	68 per serving (low).
Preparation:	Easy.
Comments:	This dip improves any party, and contains calcium, carotenes, and crucifers.

Refreshing Fruit Shake
Appetizer/snack

4 ounces nonfat or low-fat (1 percent)
 plain yogurt
1 tablespoon nonfat dry milk (leave in
 dry form)
1/4 cup buttermilk (or skim or low-fat
 milk)
1/4 cup orange juice
1/2 banana sliced (or 1 cup strawberries or
 2 ripe peaches, cut up)
2 ice cubes

Combine all ingredients in blender and whip until fruit appears well blended. Makes one 8-ounce serving.

Cost:	Inexpensive.
Calories:	186 per serving (medium).
Preparation:	Easy.
Comments:	A calcium bonanza.

Pasta e Fagioli   Soup

1/4 pound lean ground beef
Pam Cooking Spray
1 quart beef broth
1 large onion, chopped
4 fresh plum tomatoes, chopped; or
    1-ounce can peeled plum tomatoes,
    chopped and juice reserved
2 medium stalks celery, trimmed and
    sliced
2 cloves garlic, minced
1 teaspoon marjoram
1/2 teaspoon pepper
2 teaspoons chopped fresh parsley
1-pound can cannellini or small white
    beans, rinsed and drained
3/4 cup uncooked macaroni (shells, bows,
    or elbows)
Grated Parmesan cheese

Brown beef in Pam Cooking Spray and remove with slotted spoon and set aside. Place broth in Dutch oven or large kettle and add beef, onion, tomatoes (and their juice if using canned), celery, garlic, marjoram, pepper, and parsley. Cover and simmer for 45 minutes. Add beans, cover and simmer for 15 minutes. Add macaroni and simmer 6 to 8 minutes until macaroni is just tender. Sprinkle with grated Parmesan just before serving.

Serves 6.

Cost:	Inexpensive.
Calories:	254 per serving (high).
Preparation:	Easy.
Comments:	A delightful dish that also provides some carotene, fiber and calcium.

Cream of Broccoli Soup   Soup

> *1 head of fresh broccoli (cut into small*
> *   pieces)*
> *5 cups chicken broth*
> *4 tablespoons low-calorie margarine*
> *   (Promise Light)*
> *4 tablespoons flour*
> *3 cups low-fat milk*
> *Salt and pepper to taste*

Cook broccoli in chicken broth for about 20 to 25 minutes or until very tender. (Puree only broccoli in food processor.)

Melt margarine in pan and add flour. Stir constantly for 3 minutes and then add milk. Boil gently for 5 minutes; whisk or stir during cooking time. Add salt and pepper to taste. Add pureed broccoli and serve. If you wish to thin the soup, add some of the chicken broth.

Serves 6.

Cost:	Inexpensive.
Calories:	150 per serving (medium).
Preparation:	Easy.
Comments:	A dash of nutmeg is optional.

Broccoli is a crucifer that provides carotenes, fiber, and calcium. You can substitute carrots or mushrooms for broccoli to make other delicious soups. Good one day later, cold.

Lentil and Brown Rice Soup   Soup

5 cups chicken stock
3 cups water
1½ cups lentils, picked over and rinsed
1 cup brown rice
1 2-pound can tomatoes, drained,
    reserving the juice, and chopped
3 carrots, halved lengthwise and cut
    crosswise into ¼-inch pieces
1 onion, chopped
1 stalk celery, chopped
3 garlic cloves, minced
½ teaspoon crumbled dried basil
½ teaspoon crumbled dried oregano
¼ teaspoon crumbled dried thyme
1 bay leaf
½ cup minced fresh parsley leaves or 2
    tablespoons dried
2 tablespoons cider vinegar, to taste
Salt and pepper to taste

In a heavy kettle, combine the stock, 3 cups of water, lentils, rice, tomatoes, reserved tomato juice, carrots, onion, celery, garlic, basil, oregano, thyme, and the bay leaf, and bring to a boil. Simmer the mixture, covered, stirring occasionally, for 45 to 55 minutes, or until the lentils and rice are tender. Stir in the parsley, vinegar, salt and pepper, and discard the bay leaf. The soup will be thick and will thicken further as it stands. Thin the soup, if desired, with additional hot chicken stock or water. Makes about 14 cups.

Serves 6 to 12.

Cost:	Inexpensive.
Calories:	136 per serving (based on 6 servings per recipe) (medium).
Preparation:	Easy.
Comments:	Good source of fiber and carotenes.

Winter Squash Soup   Soup

Pam Cooking Spray
1 large onion, chopped
2 cloves garlic, minced
2 pounds butternut squash, peeled,
   seeded, and cut into 1-inch cubes
   (about 4 cups)
1 carrot, peeled and chopped
3 cups chicken stock or broth
1/4 teaspoon black pepper
1/4 teaspoon ground nutmeg
1 teaspoon dried basil
3/4 cup plain low-fat yogurt mixed with 2
   teaspoons corn starch

Spray the bottom of a 4- or 5-quart kettle with Pam Cooking Spray and sauté the onion and garlic for 5 minutes. Add the squash, carrot, stock, pepper, nutmeg, and basil. Cover the pot and bring to the boil. Reduce the heat and simmer for 30 minutes, or until the squash is tender. Using a food processor, blender, or food mill, puree one-third of the soup at a time. Return soup to the pan and stir in the yogurt. Reheat before serving.

Makes 6 cups.

Cost:	Inexpensive.
Calories:	152 per 1½-cup serving (medium).
Preparation:	Moderately difficult.
Comments:	Excellent source of carotenes and it tastes good.

Julienned Vegetable Salad   Salad

4 large zucchini (about 3 pounds)
4 medium carrots
1 medium green pepper
¼ medium-head red cabbage
Salt
¼ cup mayonnaise, low calorie
½ cup low-fat plain yogurt
3 teaspoons minced fresh parsley or 1
  tablespoon dried
1 teaspoon prepared mustard
1 teaspoon capers, rinsed, drained, and
  minced
½ teaspoon tarragon
Lettuce leaves

Preparation can begin early in the day, but at least 2½ hours before serving.

Cut zucchini, carrots, and green pepper into matchstick-thin strips. Finely shred cabbage to make about 1½ cups. In a large bowl, toss zucchini, carrots, green pepper, and ¾ teaspoon salt until well mixed. In a small bowl, toss red cabbage and ¼ teaspoon salt until well mixed. Cover bowls and let stand 1 hour.

Drain vegetables in large bowl by emptying into colander. Rinse vegetables well with water to remove salt and let drain for a few minutes. Rinse large bowl with water to remove salt and dry. Return vegetables to large bowl.

Repeat rinsing process with cabbage, but after draining in colander, cabbage may be placed in same bowl as vegetables.

Mix mayonnaise, yogurt, parsley, mustard, capers, and tarragon together and add to vegetable-and-cabbage mixture. Toss gently to coat with dressing. Cover and refrigerate at least 1 hour.

To serve: Line platter with lettuce leaves; arrange salad on lettuce.

Serves 8.

Cost:	Inexpensive.
Calories:	77 per serving (low).
Preparation:	Easy.
Comments:	Rich in carotenes and provides some dietary fiber.

Scandinavian Cabbage Salad   Salad

1 11-ounce can mandarin orange sections, drained
2 Delicious apples, chopped into bite-size chunks (leave peels on)
2 cups shredded green cabbage (about 1/4 of a medium head)
1 cup seedless red or green grapes
1/2 cup nonfat or low-fat plain yogurt
1/2 cup low-fat (1 percent) cottage cheese
2 tablespoons sugar
1 tablespoon lemon juice
1/4 teaspoon salt

Place orange sections, apples, cabbage, and grapes in bowl. Blend yogurt and cottage cheese in blender and transfer to small bowl. Stir in sugar, lemon juice, and salt. Stir into fruit mixture.

Serves 6.

Cost:	Inexpensive.
Calories:	97 per serving (medium).
Preparation:	Easy.
Comments:	Crucifers and calcium—and very good.

Tabbouleh (Lebanese Bean and Wheat Salad)   Salad

2 cups boiling water
1 cup extra-fine bulgur (cracked wheat)
1/2 cup cooked white beans
2 tomatoes, chopped
3 scallions, chopped
1 cup chopped parsley
1/4 cup lemon juice
1/4 cup olive oil
1 clove garlic, crushed, then minced
1/3 cup chopped fresh mint or 1
   tablespoon dried mint
1/4 teaspoon freshly ground black pepper
1/4 teaspoon salt
Romaine lettuce leaves (optional)

Pour boiling water over bulgur to cover, and allow to stand 2 hours or until wheat is light and fluffy. Drain in a fine sieve, pushing out excess water. Combine remaining ingredients, toss with bulgur, mixing well. Cover and refrigerate for at least 2 hours or overnight to allow flavors to blend thoroughly. Taste and adjust seasonings if needed. Serve chilled, alone or on romaine lettuce leaves.

Serves 4–6.

Cost:	Inexpensive.
Calories:	325 per serving (based on 4 servings per recipe) (high).
Preparation:	Moderately difficult.
Comments:	Loaded with fiber and carotene— and delicious.

Apple Cabbage Salad   Salad

4 cups shredded green cabbage
2 Winesap apples, cored and cubed. Leave
*   peel on.*
1/3 cup raisins
1/4 cup chopped green pepper
1/4 cup diet mayonnaise
1/4 cup plain low-fat yogurt
1 tablespoon apple cider vinegar
1 teaspoon prepared mustard
1/4 teaspoon each sugar and salt
Dash pepper

Combine cabbage, apples, raisins, and green pepper in bowl. Combine mayonnaise, yogurt, vinegar, mustard, sugar, salt, and pepper; pour over cabbage mixture. Toss to coat all ingredients.

Serves 6.

Cost:	Inexpensive.
Calories:	101 per serving (medium).
Preparation:	Easy.

Comments: Crucifers and fibers, plus a little
calcium. Very tasty.

White Bean and Tuna Salad   Salad

2 tablespoons red-wine vinegar
1 teaspoon Dijon-style mustard
Salt and pepper to taste
1/3 cup polyunsaturated oil or olive oil
1 16-ounce can Great Northern or white
    kidney beans, drained
2 scallions, sliced thin
3 stalks of celery, sliced thin diagonally
1/4 cup minced fresh parsley leaves or 3/4
    teaspoon dried
1 tablespoon fresh dill
1 6½-ounce can water-packed, white
    tuna, drained and flaked
5 cups shredded romaine
1 red onion, sliced thin and soaked in ice
    water

In a large bowl, whisk together the vinegar, mustard, salt,
pepper. Add the oil in a stream, whisking, and whisk the
dressing until it is emulsified. Add the beans, scallions,
celery, 2 tablespoons of the parsley, the dill, and the tuna
and toss the mixture lightly. Season the salad with salt and
pepper and chill, covered, for 1 hour. Arrange the romaine
on a platter, mound the salad on it, and garnish with the
onion, drained, and the remaining 2 tablespoons parsley.

Serves 4.

Cost: Inexpensive.
Calories: 348 per serving (high). (If used as

Preparation: main course, calorie content is
medium.)

         Easy.

Comments: Good for fiber, carotene, and
unsaturated fats.

Carrot/Cole Slaw Salad Salad

*1/2 cup mayonnaise (or reduced-calorie
  mayonnaise)*
3 tablespoons wine vinegar
Dash of sugar
1/2 head of cabbage (shredded very fine)
2 carrots (shredded very fine)

Shake mayonnaise, vinegar, and sugar well. Adjust to taste
—add more vinegar if you want it sharper. Add dressing to
cabbage and carrots and toss well.

Serves 2 to 4 (4 1-cup servings).

Cost: Inexpensive.

Calories: 112 calories per serving with
reduced-calorie mayonnaise
(medium). 236 calories per serving
with regular mayonnaise (high).

Preparation: Easy.

Comments: A great way to get carotenes,
crucifers, and some vitamin C. If
you like it, 4 good-sized portions a
week give you the weekly
recommended amounts of both
carotenes and crucifers—and it is
very tasty.

Carrot Bread with Caraway and Raisins

Grain product

2 cups all-purpose flour
3/4 teaspoon salt
1 teaspoon baking soda
1 teaspoon double-acting baking powder
1 teaspoon cinnamon
1/4 teaspoon ground allspice
1 pinch of nutmeg
1/8 teaspoon ground cloves
2 teaspoons caraway seeds
1 cup grated carrot
1 cup raisins
1/4 cup corn oil tub margarine
1 cup firmly packed brown sugar
1 large egg white, beaten lightly
1 cup buttermilk
1 tablespoon freshly grated orange rind
Pam Cooking Spray

In a bowl, combine the flour, salt, baking soda, baking powder, cinnamon, allspice, nutmeg, cloves, and the caraway seeds. Add the carrot and raisins and toss mixture to combine. In a large bowl, stir together the margarine and brown sugar, add egg white, and combine the mixture well. Stir in the buttermilk and rind. Mix well, add the flour mixture, and stir the batter until just combined. Divide the batter between two Pam-coated loaf pans, 71/4 by 31/2 by 21/4 inches, and bake in the middle of a preheated 350°F oven for 50 minutes. Then shut off oven and let cool in pans for 10 minutes in oven.

Cost: Inexpensive.
Calories: 166 per slice (medium).
Preparation: Easy.

Comments: Good source of carotene and very low in fat.

Bran Muffins

Grain product

Pam Cooking Spray
1 cup unprocessed coarse bran
1/2 cup wheat germ
1/2 cup whole wheat flour
1 tablespoon baking powder
1/2 teaspoon salt (some prefer sea salt)
1 egg
1/4 cup safflower or corn oil
1 cup low-fat milk
1/4 cup dark molasses

Preheat oven to 350°F. Spray muffin pans with Pam.

Sift together bran, wheat germ, flour, baking powder, salt. In separate bowl, beat egg and add oil, milk, molasses. Add liquid mixture to dry ingredients. Mix thoroughly. Place in pans and bake about 20 minutes. Add a cup of raisins for an interesting variation.

Makes 10 muffins.

Cost: Inexpensive.
Calories: 120 per muffin (medium).
Preparation: Easy.
Comments: High in fiber and delicious.

Oatmeal Crunch Muffins   Grain product

Streusel Mix

> 1/4 cup oats
> 1 1/2 tablespoons packed brown sugar
> 1 1/2 tablespoons chopped nuts
> 1/8 teaspoon cinnamon

Muffins

> 1/2 cup skim or low-fat milk
> 1 teaspoon lemon juice
> 1/4 cup corn oil
> 1/4 cup honey or maple syrup
> 1 egg, beaten
> 1 1/2 cups uncooked oats
> 1 cup sifted flour
> 1/2 cup chopped nuts
> 1/3 cup packed brown sugar
> 1 tablespoon baking powder

To make streusel mix, pulse together ingredients in food processor (or chop nuts and mix together).

To make muffins, combine lemon juice, milk, oil, egg, and honey or maple syrup. Mix dry ingredients together and make a well in the center. Pour in liquid ingredients, mixing by hand just until dry ingredients are moistened. Place about a tablespoon of muffin batter in the bottom of each paper-lined baking cup. Sprinkle a small amount of streusel mix on the batter. Use remaining batter to fill cups three-quarters full. Sprinkle with streusel mix. Bake in preheated hot oven (400°F) for 15 to 18 minutes or until golden brown. Variation: Add 1/2 cup raisins.

Serves 12.

Cost:	Inexpensive (it is more economical if made with honey, as maple syrup is expensive).
Calories:	220 each (high).
Preparation:	Easy.
Comments:	These muffins are moist and delicious. Each provides about 2 grams of dietary fiber, predominantly oat fiber, which may be helpful in lowering blood cholesterol levels.

Whole Wheat Popovers   Grain product

1 cup whole wheat flour
1 teaspoon light brown sugar
1 cup skim or low-fat milk
1 teaspoon corn oil
1 egg plus 2 egg whites
Butter-flavored Pam Cooking Spray

Combine flour, sugar, milk, and oil. Mix with a spoon. Beat eggs by hand and fold gently into flour mixture. (Let eggs stand at room temperature a couple of hours before using.)

Spray muffin tins well with butter-flavored Pam and fill three-quarters full with mixture. Place in cold oven. Turn on oven to 425°F. Bake for 30 minutes, then reduce oven to 350°F for an additional 10 minutes.

When popovers are done, take straight pin and gently prick top to allow steam to escape.

Makes 10 popovers.

Cost:	Inexpensive.
Calories:	65 per popover (low).

Preparation: Easy.
Comments: Marvelous taste and lots of fiber.

Zucchini Bread
Grain product

Pam Cooking Spray
2 cups unbleached white flour
1 cup minus 2 tablespoons whole wheat
flour
1 cup sugar
3/4 cup walnuts, chopped
1 teaspoon each of salt, baking powder,
and baking soda
2 eggs plus 2 egg whites
2/3 cup corn or safflower oil
2 cups grated, unpeeled zucchini
2 teaspoons grated lemon peel
1 teaspoon cinnamon

Preheat oven to 350°F. Spray two 9-by-5-inch loaf pans with Pam Cooking Spray. In a large bowl, with fork, mix flour, sugar, walnuts, salt, baking powder, and baking soda. In a medium bowl, with fork, beat eggs slightly, stir in oil, zucchini, lemon peel, and cinnamon. Stir into flour mixture just until flour is moistened and spread batter evenly in pans. Bake 1 hour or until toothpick inserted in center comes out clean. Cool in pans for 10 minutes before removing.

Makes 2 loaves.

Cost: Inexpensive.
Calories: 250 per slice (8 slices per loaf)
(high).
Preparation: Easy.

Comments: Fiber, some carotene, and very tasty.

All-in-One Baked Brown Rice with Vegetables

Grain product

1 cup brown rice
2½ cups chicken broth
1 large onion, minced
2 carrots, shredded
¾ tablespoon oregano
3 to 4 sprigs chopped parsley
⅛ tablespoon ground pepper
2 tablespoons margarine
1 clove garlic, minced fine
¾ tablespoon thyme
1 cup defrosted green peas (optional)

Place all ingredients in a casserole. Mix. Cover with light lid or aluminum foil. Bake at 350°F for approximately 1 hour.

Serves 6.

Cost: Inexpensive.
Calories: 248 per serving (with peas) (low).
Preparation: Easy.
Comments: Lots of fiber and carotene and it tastes good.

Bulgur Pilaf with Nuts

Grain product

1 small onion, sliced thin
1 tablespoon margarine
½ cup bulgur

¾ cup chicken broth (canned)
3 to 4 tablespoons chopped, unsalted, dry-
  roasted cashews
Approximately 1 tablespoon thinly sliced
  scallions (include green top)

Cook onion in margarine slowly until softened. Stir in bulgur, cooking mixture for 1 minute while stirring. Add broth and bring to boil. Cover, reduce heat, and cook until liquid is absorbed (approximately 10 minutes). Stir with fork and sprinkle pilaf with nuts and scallions.

Serves 2.

Cost:	Inexpensive.
Calories:	325 per serving (medium).
Preparation:	Easy.
Comments:	Nice change from rice and pasta. High in fiber.

Savory Linguine with Broccoli and Herbs

Meatless main dish

¼ cup unsalted tub margarine
1 tablespoon olive oil
1½ pints cherry tomatoes, stems removed
1 cup chicken broth or stock
2 to 3 large cloves of garlic, minced
Red pepper flakes to taste
¼ teaspoon sweet basil
3 stalks fresh broccoli cut into flowerets,
  about 6 cups
12 ounces linguine
¼ cup freshly grated Romano cheese
¼ cup chopped fresh parsley

Melt 1/4 cup of margarine and 1 tablespoon of olive oil over moderate heat in a medium-sized skillet. Add the tomatoes and sauté, stirring often, for 2 minutes. Add the broth, garlic, pepper flakes, and basil, and cook 25 minutes longer, until tomatoes are tender but still hold their shape. Meanwhile, boil water for linguine and cook according to package directions. Add the broccoli to linguine during the last 3 minutes of cooking time. After draining linguine and broccoli thoroughly, toss with tomatoes, broth, etc. Top with Romano cheese, fresh parsley and serve.

Serves 4.

Cost:	Inexpensive.
Calories:	522 per serving (high).
Preparation:	Easy.
Comments:	Crucifers, fibers, and calcium; and the garlic may be good for the heart.

Meatless Taco Casserole
Meatless main dish

1 large onion, coarsely chopped
1 clove garlic, minced
1 cup coarsely chopped fresh mushrooms
   (about 1/4 pound)
1/3 cup chopped fresh parsley
1/4 cup finely chopped sweet green pepper
1 tablespoon vegetable oil
2 cans (16 ounces each) pinto beans, well
   drained
1/2 cup tomato sauce
2 to 3 tablespoons chopped green chilies,
   canned, or to taste
21/4 teaspoons chili powder
1/2 teaspoon ground cumin (optional)

1/8 teaspoon ground celery seed
1/8 teaspoon black pepper
10 to 11 regular-size unsalted nacho chips
1/2 cup shredded Cheddar cheese
1/2 cup shredded part-skim mozzarella
2 medium-size tomatoes, cored and
  coarsely chopped
11/4 cups shredded iceberg lettuce (1/4
  head)
1/2 cup thinly sliced green onions with
  tops (optional)

Preheat oven to very slow (275°F). Sauté onion, garlic, mushrooms, parsley, and green pepper in oil in large skillet until soft, about 7 minutes.

Coarsely mash pinto beans with potato masher (or fork). Add beans to skillet, along with tomato sauce, green chilies, chili powder, cumin, celery seed, and pepper. Cook, stirring frequently, 10 minutes, or until almost all moisture has evaporated. Spread half the nacho chips in bottom of shallow 11/2-quart casserole. Spoon bean mixture in even layer over nacho chips. Sprinkle top of casserole with cheese and remaining nacho chips.

Bake in preheated, warm oven (275°F) for 4 to 5 minutes, or until cheese melts. Sprinkle tomatoes, lettuce, and chopped green onions, if using, over cheese.

Serves 6.

Cost:	Inexpensive.
Calories:	392 per serving (medium).
Preparation:	Moderately difficult.
Comments:	Very good for weight control plus plenty of fiber. Provides a lot of carotenes and at least 250 milligrams of calcium per serving.

Meatless Chili

Meatless main dish

1 pound dried pinto beans
Pam Cooking Spray
2 onions, chopped
2 cloves garlic, chopped
1 carrot, sliced
1 green pepper, chopped
1 zucchini, sliced
2 teaspoons chili powder
1/2 teaspoon cumin
1 teaspoon salt (optional)
1 1/2 teaspoon oregano
1 cup chicken or beef stock (or broth)
1 cup chopped tomatoes (fresh or canned)
*1/3 cup bulgur (cracked wheat) or rice or 1
    cup corn*

Cover beans with 3 inches of water and let soak overnight or boil for 3 minutes and let stand for 1 hour. Drain. Add 6 cups of water to kettle and cook beans until tender but not mushy. In a large pot, sauté onions and garlic in the Pam Cooking Spray until wilted. Add carrot to onions and continue cooking for 3 to 5 minutes. Add peppers, zucchini, the seasonings, and cook for 5 more minutes. Add stock, tomatoes, beans, and bulgur to the vegetables. Simmer over a low flame until the bulgur has absorbed some of the liquid and flavors of the herbs and spices (approximately 15 minutes), stirring occasionally. Add more water if chili becomes too thick. May be served on rice.

Serves 8.

Cost:	Inexpensive.
Calories:	211 calories per serving (based on 6 servings per recipe) (low).
Preparation:	Moderately difficult.

Comments: Lots of fiber and carotenes; good for
              weight control.

Fish Fiesta   Seafood

1 pound fish fillets (flounder, red snapper,
  scrod)
1/4 teaspoon pepper
1 small onion, thinly sliced and
  separated into rings
1 tomato, cut into chunks
1 tablespoon lime (or lemon) juice
1 tablespoon chopped parsley
1 teaspoon oregano
Pam Cooking Spray
Lime or lemon wedges

If fish fillets are large, cut into 5 or 6 serving pieces.
Arrange fish in ungreased square baking dish, 8 by 8 by 2
inches; sprinkle with pepper. Top with onion, tomato, lime
(or lemon) juice, parsley, and oregano. Spray with Pam for
just under 1 second. Cover and cook in 375°F oven for 15
minutes. Uncover and cook until fish flakes easily with
fork, about 15 minutes longer. Garnish with lime or lemon
wedges.

Serves 4.

Cost: Moderate to expensive.
Calories: 276 per serving (medium, if flounder
               used; low, if red snapper served).
Preparation: Easy.
Comments: This is a very tasty dish; the cost
               and calorie content vary, depending
               on which fish fillet you choose.

Creole Fillets à la New Orleans   Seafood

*1 pound flounder or red snapper fillet
  (other white fish may be substituted)
1 medium tomato, chopped
1/2 small green pepper, chopped (about 1/4
  cup)
3 tablespoons lemon juice
Pam Cooking Spray
1/4 cup white wine
1 teaspoon salt
1 teaspoon grated onion
1/2 teaspoon dried basil leaves
1/8 teaspoon coarsely ground black pepper
2 drops red pepper sauce
Green pepper rings (optional)
Tomato wedges (optional)*

If fish fillets are large, cut into 4 serving pieces. Place fish
in an oblong baking dish, 13 1/2 by 9 by 2 inches, that has
been sprayed with Pam. Mix remaining ingredients; spoon
onto fish. Cook, uncovered, in 400°F oven until fish flakes
easily with fork, about 10 minutes. Garnish with green
pepper rings and tomato wedges if desired.

Serves 4.

Cost:	Moderate to expensive.
Calories:	262 per serving (medium, if flounder used; low, if red snapper served).
Preparation:	Easy.
Comments:	Cost depends on type of fish fillet chosen.

Fish Fillets in Soy Marinade   Seafood

Marinade

> 1 cup soy sauce
> 1/2 cup water
> 1/2 cup dry white wine
> 1 clove garlic
> 1 1/2 tablespoons sliced fresh ginger
> 2 tablespoons lemon juice

Fish

> 1 pound of any of the following: cod,
>   butterfish, sole, or similar fish

> *Pam Cooking Spray*
> *Lemon slices*

Marinate fish fillets for a minimum of 4 hours, turning once.

Spray casserole lightly with Pam. Place fillets in casserole and pour in enough marinade to cover bottom of dish. (Refrigerate leftover marinade for use a second time.) Place on center rack in preheated 350°F oven for 20 to 25 minutes. Serve with lemon slices.

Serves 4.

Cost:	Moderate.
Calories:	277 per serving (medium).
Preparation:	Easy.
Comments:	Cost is dependent on type of fillet used and area of the country. Low in saturated fats.

Poached Fish and Vegetables   Seafood

*4 small fish fillets, approximately 1
  pound (flounder, sole)*
Lemon juice to taste
2 teaspoons grated Parmesan cheese
2 tomatoes, chopped
1 small zucchini, sliced paper-thin
Dash of salt
1 green pepper, diced fine (optional)
1 small onion, diced fine
1/2 teaspoon oregano
1/4 cup white wine or fish or chicken stock

Sprinkle fish with lemon juice and grated cheese. Roll up
and set aside on plate. In skillet, simmer tomatoes,
zucchini, salt, pepper, onion, and oregano in wine for 3
minutes. Place rolled fish in vegetable mixture. Cover and
cook over low heat for 5 to 7 minutes until fish flakes.

Serves 4.

Cost:	Moderate.
Calories:	264 per serving (medium).
Preparation:	Easy.
Comments:	Cost is dependent on type of fish used. Good for weight control; if blood pressure elevated or borderline, or if you are having trouble with weight loss, forget the salt.

Swordfish on Skewers   Seafood

2 pounds swordfish
3 tablespoons lemon juice

Olive Oil Pam Cooking Spray
2 tablespoons melted margarine
1/2 teaspoon onion salt
1/2 teaspoon paprika
Grind fresh pepper to taste
2 bay leaves
2 tablespoons minced parsley

Remove skin from swordfish and cut into 1½-inch cubes. Spray fish on both sides with Pam and marinate all day (or 6 hours) in mixture of other above ingredients, coating fish well. Place on skewers alternating with chunks of onion, peppers, and tomatoes, if desired, and place skewers under broiler or on a barbecue, turning and basting with remaining marinade. Spray with Pam before cooking and each time you turn fish. Cook approximately 10 minutes.

Serves 6.

Cost:	Expensive.
Calories:	360 per serving (medium).
Preparation:	Easy.
Comments:	Swordfish is outrageously expensive in most areas of the country, but it certainly tastes good and it's low in saturated fats.

Shrimp Broiled in Herbs   Seafood

2 pounds large shrimp
Olive Oil Pam Cooking Spray
4 to 5 cloves of fresh garlic, minced fine
2 to 3 tablespoons chopped parsley
1/8 teaspoon red pepper flakes
1/2 teaspoon oregano

2 tablespoons whole wheat fine bread
crumbs
Salt and pepper to taste
Juice of 1 large lemon

Shell and clean shrimp, leaving tail on. Rinse in cold water and drain well. Spray shrimp well on all sides with Pam. Mix all other above ingredients. Add shrimp, tossing about until coated with marinade. Cover and place in refrigerator for 3 to 4 hours. Line broiler pan with heavy-duty foil and lay shrimp on it. Spray shrimp again with Pam and pour remaining marinade over before putting under broiler. Place under very hot (preheated) broiler, 3 to 4 inches from heat, and broil 5 to 6 minutes, or less. Keep close watch; do not overcook. Not necessary to turn shrimp. Serve over brown rice, linguine, or wild rice.

Serves 4 to 5.

Cost:	Expensive.
Calories:	420 per serving (based on 5 servings per recipe) (medium).
Preparation:	Easy.
Comments:	It tastes great, but it is a bit pricey.

Herb-Baked Fish   Seafood

3/4 cup unflavored whole wheat bread
crumbs
3 large garlic cloves, minced
1/2 teaspoon thyme
1/2 teaspoon sage
Salt and pepper
6 medium fish fillets (sole, flounder)
1 lemon

*2 tablespoons corn oil or safflower tub
    margarine
1/4 cup dry white wine
2 tablespoons chopped fresh parsley*

Preheat oven to 400°F. In a small bowl, mix together bread crumbs, garlic, thyme, sage, and salt and pepper to taste. Set aside. Rinse the fillets of fish under cold water. Pat dry with paper towels. Arrange in large, shallow, oiled baking dish, overlapping if necessary. Squeeze the juice of one lemon over the fillets. Scatter the bread crumb mixture over the fish. Cut the margarine into small pieces and distribute evenly over the crumbs. Drizzle wine over fillets and sprinkle with parsley. Bake for 20 minutes or until fish flakes easily with a fork. Place under broiler for a couple of minutes to brown top—watch carefully.

Serves 6.

Cost:	Moderate to expensive.
Calories:	374 per serving (medium).
Preparation:	Easy.
Comments:	Cost depends on type of fish chosen. Good for unsaturated fats.

Four for Red Snapper   Seafood

*4 small red snapper fillets (approximately
    1 pound) in pan lined with foil
Promise Light margarine
Salt and pepper
Pinch of ground thyme
1/2 cup finely chopped celery
1/2 red or green pepper, finely chopped
2 tablespoons chopped parsley*

1 small onion, sliced thin
2 small garlic cloves, minced

Rub fillets with margarine. Add salt and pepper to taste. Sprinkle fish with thyme, celery, red or green pepper, and parsley.

In separate saucepan, heat approximately 2 to 3 tablespoons margarine with the onion and garlic. Sauté until soft but not brown.

Place this over fish and bake in 325°F oven approximately 30 minutes.

Serves 4.

Cost:	Expensive.
Calories:	209 per serving (low).
Preparation:	Easy.
Comments:	Usually with red snapper, the simpler the preparation, the better. Too bad this fish is so expensive in many areas of the country.

Paula's Party Sea Legs Salad   Seafood

2 pounds sea legs
3/4 cup diet mayonnaise
3/4 cup Heinz Chili Sauce
Knorr's Swiss All Purpose Seasoning to
*   taste*

Sea legs come frozen in packages, or you can buy them by the pound at your fish market. Drain thoroughly, whether fresh or frozen, and squeeze out all water.

Mix the mayonnaise, chili sauce, and seasoning. Then taste, adjust, and toss in a bowl with sea legs. Place on lettuce leaves and surround with tomatoes, radishes, carrots, and peppers.

Serves 6 to 8.

Cost:	Inexpensive.
Calories:	185 per serving (low, if used as a main dish).
Preparation:	Easy.
Comments:	I don't know who Paula is, but the sea legs taste good.

Sole Smothered in Lemon   Seafood

*4 pieces of sole or 2 large fillets (about 1
    pound)*
1/4 cup skim or 1 percent low-fat milk
Salt and pepper to taste
1 large lemon
3 tablespoons fresh chopped parsley
1 tablespoon capers, drained
Pam Cooking Spray
4 tablespoons margarine

Soak fish in milk for about 1 hour. Add salt and pepper.

Peel lemon so only flesh remains, discard seeds and chop. Chop parsley. Drain capers.

Heat Pam in large pan, adding 1 tablespoon of margarine. Remove fish from milk. Dip into seasoned flour, shaking off excess. Place fish in hot oil and brown on both sides (takes about 5 minutes). Transfer to hot platter and keep warm. Heat remaining margarine, add lemon and capers, and pour over fish. Top with parsley and serve at once.

Serves 4.

Cost:	Moderate to expensive.
Calories:	477 per serving (medium).
Preparation:	Easy.
Comments:	This is a marvelous fish dish. If lemon sole is used, it is more expensive. Low in saturated fat.

Monkfish Pizza Style Seafood

1½ to 2 pounds monkfish, cut into 2-inch
  cubes
1 8-ounce can crushed plum tomatoes
½ to 1 teaspoon oregano
2 tablespoons finely chopped parsley
1 large garlic clove, finely minced
Salt and freshly ground pepper to taste
Pinch of crushed red pepper
¼ cup grated Parmesan cheese
Pam Cooking Spray

Place monkfish in casserole. Cover with layer of tomatoes. Sprinkle with oregano, parsley, garlic, salt and pepper, red pepper, and grated cheese. Spray with Pam for just under 1 second.

Place, uncovered, in preheated 350°F oven, until fish becomes milk-white and is fork-tender (about 30 to 35 minutes). This dish is wonderful served on bed of brown rice or linguine.

Serves 4.

Cost:	Moderate.
Calories:	322 per serving (medium).
Preparation:	Easy.
Comments:	Provides protein, beta-carotene, and some calcium (140 milligrams per

serving). Tastes great, but watch
that you don't overdo the red
pepper.

Country Baked Chicken

Poultry

*1 3¼-pound chicken, cut up into pieces
    and skin removed*
8 small new potatoes with skins
5 carrots, cut into 2-inch slices
8 small boiling onions, peeled
1 bell pepper, sliced
¾ cup dry white wine
¾ cup chicken broth
*1½ tablespoons corn or safflower oil tub
    margarine*
Salt and pepper to taste
2 tablespoons of basil
3 cloves garlic, minced
½ pound fresh mushrooms, halved
Pam Cooking Spray
½ cup Parmesan cheese
Paprika

Place chicken, potatoes, carrots, onions, bell pepper, wine,
and broth into rectangular pan. Dot chicken with
margarine, add salt, pepper, and basil. Bake uncovered at
400°F for 30 minutes, basting several times. In separate
pan, sauté garlic and mushrooms in Pam Cooking Spray
and add to roasting pan after 30 minutes of baking.
Sprinkle chicken with Parmesan cheese and paprika. Cover
and cook an additional 30 to 40 minutes at 350°F.

Serves 8.

Cost:	Moderate.
Calories:	595 per serving (high).
Preparation:	Moderately difficult.
Comments:	Recipe can be doubled by using either two chickens or one chicken and extra thighs and legs. Increase all other ingredients accordingly. Rich in carotene.

Braised Turkey Legs Supreme   Poultry

1/2 cup all-purpose flour
1 teaspoon salt
1 teaspoon oregano
1/2 teaspoon pepper
4 turkey drumsticks (wings may also be used)
Pam Cooking Spray
2 large onions, chopped fine
2 cloves garlic, minced
1 14 1/2-ounce can chicken broth
1/2 cup dry red wine
2 bay leaves
1 teaspoon thyme
1 teaspoon rosemary

Combine flour, salt, oregano, and pepper in a plastic bag. Dredge turkey in flour mixture, shake off excess, and set aside leftover mixture.

Spray large frying pan with Pam. Brown turkey pieces on all sides, and transfer to casserole. Add onions and garlic to frying pan and cook until soft. Stir in broth, wine, bay leaves, thyme, and rosemary. Pour mixture over turkey legs in casserole and bake in 350°F oven for 2 1/2 to 3 hours. Transfer legs to serving platter.

Blend leftover flour with equal amount of water and stir into pan juices until thickened. Spoon over turkey. Serve with brown rice or noodles.

Serves 4.

Cost:	Inexpensive.
Calories:	437 per serving (medium).
Preparation:	Easy.
Comments:	An olfactory delight—and low-fat.

Chicken Cassoulet   Poultry

1½ *pounds boneless, skinless chicken (or*
    turkey), a combination of breast and
    thigh meat, cut into 1-inch cubes
6 *garlic cloves, crushed with flat side of*
    knife blade, then minced
1 *teaspoon ground thyme*
Pinch of ground allspice
Pam Cooking Spray
2 *cups chopped onion*
1 *16-ounce can whole tomatoes, cut in*
    quarters, saving juice
½ *teaspoon dried rosemary*
2 *bay leaves*
1 *tablespoon chopped fresh parsley or 1*
    teaspoon dried parsley
½ *cup dry white wine*
2 *16-ounce cans of white or Great*
    Northern beans, rinsed and drained
1½ *cups chicken stock*
½ *cup dry bread crumbs*

Toss chicken cubes with ½ teaspoon of minced garlic and the thyme and allspice. Let stand 1 hour (or refrigerate overnight). In a large, heavy, deep skillet, heat the Pam and sauté chicken pieces until light brown, about 3 minutes on each side. Remove chicken with slotted spoon and set aside. Sauté onion and remainder of garlic in skillet until golden. Add tomatoes and their juice, rosemary, bay leaves, parsley, and wine. Reduce the heat to low and simmer the mixture, stirring frequently, about 10 minutes. Spread half of the beans over the bottom of a large, deep casserole. Cover the beans with the chicken pieces to form another layer. Spoon half the tomato and onion mixture over the chicken, then add the remaining beans in another layer. Spoon remaining tomato mixture over them. Pour in 1 cup chicken stock and sprinkle with bread crumbs. Bake at 375°F for 45 minutes, then pour the remaining stock around the edges of the casserole to keep from getting dry. Bake another 15 minutes.

Serves 6 to 8.

Cost:	Moderate.
Calories:	485 per serving (based on 6 servings per recipe) (medium).
Preparation:	Moderately difficult.
Comments:	The chicken is low-fat if you remove the skin, and the beans add fiber. High in carotenes. Provides considerable dietary fiber.

Succulent Chicken Breasts in Hollandaise

Poultry

1½ pounds boneless chicken breasts
3 cups of cooked brown or wild rice
½ medium-head cauliflower, cut into
    flowerets and steamed for 3 minutes
½ cup shredded Cheddar cheese

Poach 6 boned chicken breasts in hot water until partially done (do not overcook).

Place breasts on top of cooked brown rice or wild rice. Place cauliflower around chicken and rice. Cover all with hollandaise sauce and sprinkle lightly with Cheddar cheese. Place in preheated 400°F oven for about 20 minutes.

Serves 6.

Hollandaise Sauce

> *2 egg yolks*
> *1 tablespoon lemon juice*
> *1/2 teaspoon salt*
> *Dash of cayenne*
> *1/3 cup margarine*

Place egg yolks, lemon juice, salt, and cayenne in blender. Switch on for a few seconds and then off. Heat margarine to boiling point. Turn blender on and pour margarine in while machine is running. Turn off as soon as margarine is added.

Makes 1/2 cup.

Cost:	Moderate to expensive.
Calories:	464 calories per serving (including sauce) (medium).
Preparation:	Moderately difficult.
Comments:	A solid chicken recipe; the hollandaise adds a lot. Must remove skins. Hollandaise is high in cholesterol, so this dish is only for those with cholesterol levels under 200 to 210. Also provides fiber and crucifers.

Garnished Chicken with Peanuts, Carrots, and Rice

Poultry

1/2 cup brown rice
Pam Cooking Spray
1/2 pound boneless, skinless chicken
    breast, cut into half-inch pieces
3/4 cup dry white wine
1 cup canned chicken broth
2 carrots, cut into half-inch pieces
16 scallions (white portion), cut into half-
    inch pieces
1 tablespoon soy sauce
2 teaspoons fresh lime juice (or to taste)
1/4 cup chopped dry-roasted unsalted
    peanuts
1/4 cup thinly sliced scallion greens
Cayenne pepper to taste
Salt and pepper to taste
Thin slices of lime for garnish

Add rice to large saucepan of boiling salted water for 15 minutes. Drain and bring 1/3 cup water to boil in small pan and add partially cooked rice. Cook, covered, over low heat for approximately 15 minutes more or until tender and all water is absorbed. Keep rice covered until ready to use.

In heavy skillet, heat the Pam and brown the chicken for 2 to 3 minutes or until it is springy to the touch. Transfer to small bowl.

Add 1/4 cup of wine to the skillet. Stir, scraping up the brown bits. Add the remaining 1/2 cup of wine, broth, and carrots, and cook, covered, for 5 minutes. Add the scallions, cover, and cook over moderate heat for another 15 minutes. Stir in the chicken, soy sauce, and lime juice.

In large bowl, combine rice, peanuts, scallion greens, chicken mixture, cayenne, and salt and pepper. Toss mixture well and transfer to heated dish. Garnish with lime slices.

Serves 2.

Cost:	Moderate.
Calories:	650 per serving (high).
Preparation:	Easy.
Comments:	High-calorie, low-fat; the peanuts, scallions, and lime are a great combination and provide plenty of carotenes. Good source of dietary fiber.

Savory Marinated Chicken Parmesan   Poultry

1 cup plain nonfat yogurt
6 tablespoons lemon juice
2 tablespoons Dijon mustard
5 garlic cloves, minced
1/2 teaspoon salt
1/2 teaspoon dried oregano
1/2 teaspoon dried marjoram
1/4 teaspoon dried thyme
1/8 teaspoon black pepper
1 2- to 3-pound chicken; remove skin and
   cut into 8 serving pieces
1/2 cup unflavored whole wheat bread
   crumbs
1/2 cup grated Parmesan cheese
1/8 teaspoon cayenne pepper
1/4 cup Promise Light margarine, melted

Combine yogurt, lemon juice, mustard, garlic, salt, and herbs in bowl. Add pepper to taste. Add the chicken pieces and stir to coat them with the marinade. Let chicken marinate, covered, in refrigerator for at least 2 hours, preferably overnight.

In a plastic or paper bag, combine bread crumbs, Parmesan cheese, cayenne, and pepper. Drain the chicken pieces and shake each one in the bread crumb mixture until well coated.

Arrange the pieces in a well-oiled baking dish, leaving about 1 inch between them. Chill for 1 hour. Drizzle the melted margarine over the chicken and bake in a preheated oven at 350°F for 40 minutes.

Serves 6 to 8.

Cost:	Moderate.
Calories:	351 (based on 8 servings per recipe) (medium).
Preparation:	Moderately difficult.
Comments:	The extra preparation time is worth it; contains a modest amount of calcium.

Honey-Orange Chicken   Poultry

1 large broiler, split
Salt and pepper
1/4 cup honey
1/2 cup concentrated orange juice

Lay chicken pieces skin side down in broiling pan. Salt and pepper each piece. Mix the honey and orange juice in a small pan. Heat carefully over low flame, stirring until well mixed, approximately 1 minute.

Coat chicken with orange-honey mixture and place on lowest rung of broiler—farthest from the flame. Cook 35 to 40 minutes, basting if necessary. Turn chicken skin side up.

Coat well with remaining orange-honey mix and continue cooking, watching and basting, for another 20 to 30 minutes. Be careful not to burn—should be glazed and deeply browned. If this occurs before chicken is fully cooked, remove chicken from under broiler and finish the cooking process in a 400°F oven.

Serve with brown rice covered with pan drippings.

Serves 6 to 8.

Cost:	Moderate.
Calories:	313 per serving (based on 6 servings per recipe) (medium).
Preparation:	Easy.
Comments:	This is a very good chicken dish. The rice adds fiber. To reduce saturated fat and calories, remove chicken skin.

Chicken Wrapped in Mustard Sauce   Poultry

1 broiler, split (or small chicken,
  quartered), skin removed
Dijon mustard (enough to coat)
1/2 cup white wine
1/2 cup evaporated skim milk
Chopped parsley for garnish

Preheat oven to 350°F. Coat both sides of chicken with Dijon mustard. Allow to sit, covered, in baking pan for 1 hour at room temperature before cooking. Place chicken and white wine in pan and bake in oven for 1 hour. Remove juices from cooking pan and bring to a boil. Add evaporated milk. Cook, stirring, for about 5 minutes. Pour over chicken. Toss on some chopped parsley. Serve with brown rice or bulgur wheat.

Serves 4.

Cost:	Inexpensive to moderate.
Calories:	338 per serving (medium).
Preparation:	Easy.
Comments:	Tasty, low in fat, provides some calcium (138 milligrams per serving).

Veal Piccata   Meat

*8 very thin slices of veal (approximately 1
   pound)*
1/2 cup flour
Salt and white pepper to taste
1/3 cup vegetable oil
2 or 3 lemons
*2 to 3 tablespoons finely chopped fresh
   parsley*

Dust each slice of veal very lightly with flour mixed with salt and pepper. Shake off excess. Heat some of the oil in large frying pan until hot. Sauté veal very quickly on both sides. When lightly browned, squeeze with fresh lemon and dot with parsley. Transfer to warm oven and repeat steps until all the veal is cooked. Serve at once.

Serves 4.

Cost:	Expensive.
Calories:	438 per serving (medium).
Preparation:	Easy.

Comments: There is no better veal dish than this. Unfortunately, veal is expensive.

Ginger Veal Meatloaf Delight

Meat

2 pounds gound veal (use steer veal)
Salt and pepper
1 cup finely chopped onions
1 cup finely chopped celery
1 large clove garlic, finely minced
Pam Cooking Spray
4 slices white bread, cubed, with crusts
    removed
1/2 cup skim milk, warmed
1 egg, slightly beaten
1 tablespoon finely minced fresh ginger

Add salt and pepper to taste to ground veal. In a separate pan, sauté onions, celery, and garlic in Pam Cooking Spray. Cook until tender; do not brown.

Soak cubed white bread in warm skim milk.

Add egg and ginger to veal. Now add all remaining ingredients to meat, mix thoroughly, and place in loaf pan. Bake in 425°F oven for approximately 1 hour. Serve with fresh tomato sauce or Prego's tomato sauce with fresh sweet red peppers.

Serves 6.

Cost:	Expensive.
Calories:	425 per serving (medium).
Preparation:	Easy.
Comments:	The more you mix ingredients, the finer-grained the meatloaf, and it is

wonderful; try slicing it very thin and use like pâté.

Calcium-Stuffed Potatoes   Vegetable

1 large baked potato
1/4 cup part-skim ricotta cheese
1 teaspoon grated Parmesan cheese
Dash of salt and pepper
1/2 cup lightly steamed broccoli flowerets
1 teaspoon of Promise Light margarine

Slice potato in half. Remove inside of potato carefully and mash. Add cheeses, salt, and pepper and mix gently. Stuff back in potato skins, place in warm oven and, when very hot, cover tops with broccoli seasoned with a little margarine and sprinkle of Parmesan cheese.

Serves 1.

Cost:	Inexpensive.
Calories:	263 per serving (high).
Preparation:	Easy.
Comments:	Crucifers, calcium, and fiber; a pretty good combination.

Lemon-Soy Broccoli   Vegetable

2 bunches broccoli
6 tablespoons margarine (or olive oil or
*   peanut oil to taste)*
3 tablespoons total lemon juice and soy
*   sauce mixed in equal parts (or to taste)*

Remove the flowerets from broccoli and cut stems into thin slices crosswise (or reserve stems for another use). Stir-fry broccoli pieces in margarine in a wok or deep skillet over high heat, adding splashes of the lemon-soy mixture to taste. Cook only until the flowerets are just tender. Adjust seasonings and serve.

Serves 6.

Cost:	Inexpensive.
Calories:	129 per serving (medium).
Preparation:	Easy.
Comments:	This is a great way to serve broccoli, and it provides a lot nutritionally—fiber, cruciferous vegetables, and carotenes.

Marinated Vegetable Treat   Vegetable

1 package garlic salad dressing mix
Corn, safflower, or olive oil
1/4 cup grated Parmesan cheese
Freshly ground black pepper
1 cup raw cauliflowerets
1 cup small-capped raw mushrooms
1 cup cherry tomatoes
1 cup raw broccoli flowerets and shaved
  stem pieces

Prepare salad dressing according to package directions, using one of the above-mentioned oils. Add Parmesan cheese and freshly ground black pepper to taste. Pour over vegetables and marinate overnight in refrigerator.

Serves 8.

Cost:	Inexpensive.
Calories:	Approximately 200 per serving (medium).
Preparation:	Easy.
Comments:	Crucifers, carotenes, plus some calcium, and it's delicious.

Ginger Broccoli
Vegetable

Pam Cooking Spray
1 tablespoon minced fresh ginger
3 shallots, minced, or 1 scallion, minced
6 cups broccoli flowerets
1/2 cup chicken stock
2 teaspoons low-sodium soy sauce
2 teaspoons rice wine vinegar
1 teaspoon cornstarch

Heat Pam Cooking Spray in large skillet or wok. Add ginger and shallots. Sauté until shallots are wilted. Add the broccoli and stir-fry for 1 minute. Mix together the chicken stock, soy sauce, vinegar, and cornstarch, and pour over broccoli. Cover and cook until broccoli is tender but still crisp. Serve hot or cold.

Serves 4 to 6.

Cost:	Inexpensive.
Calories:	80 per serving (based on 4 servings per recipe) (low).
Preparation:	Easy.
Comments:	A great way to serve broccoli, one of the best of the crucifers (plus fiber and carotenes).

Brussels Sprouts Supreme   Vegetable

4 cups Brussels sprouts
4 tablespoons sherry vinegar
4 tablespoons maple syrup (pure)
1 tablespoons Dijon-style mustard
1/2 cup walnut oil
Salt and pepper to taste
Pinch of nutmeg
1/2 cup walnuts

Cut an *x* on bottom of each Brussels sprout. Steam until tender but firm. Whisk vinegar, syrup, and mustard together, gradually adding oil. Season with salt and pepper and nutmeg. Toss sherry vinegar, nuts, and Brussels sprouts together to mix well.

Serves 4 to 6.

Cost:	Moderate.
Calories:	306 per serving (based on 4 servings per recipe) (high).
Preparation:	Easy.
Comments:	A very tasty crucifer recipe indeed, plus some fiber.

Brussels Sprouts with Onions   Vegetable

1 pint Brussels sprouts
Salt to taste
Pam Cooking Spray
1/4 cup finely chopped onions

Boil Brussels sprouts about 10 to 12 minutes. Drain. Add a pinch of salt to drained sprouts, if desired. Spray a separate pan with Pam and heat. Add onions and cook until soft.

Add drained Brussels sprouts. Continue to cook about 5 minutes, shaking pan a little, and serve.

Serves 3.

Cost:	Inexpensive.
Calories:	110 per serving (medium).
Preparation:	Easy.
Comments:	Brussels sprouts are, of course, one of the cruciferous vegetables. Ease of preparation is a major virtue of this recipe. Provides carotene and some fiber.

Hungarian Noodle Cabbage Dish   Vegetable

4 medium onions, sliced
1 large head of green cabbage, shredded
3 tablespoons Wesson oil
3 tablespoons margarine
1 1-pound package medium noodles
Salt and pepper

Sauté onions and cabbage together in large skillet in oil and margarine, combined. Cook noodles (not too soft) and drain dry. Mix cabbage with noodles. Add salt and pepper to taste. Add margarine if too dry.

Serves 6.

Cost:	Inexpensive.
Calories:	352 per serving (medium).
Preparation:	Easy.
Comments:	Cabbage is one of the crucifers, and this is good way to prepare it. Also provides some fiber.

Barbara's Festive Cauliflower in Cheese Soufflé

Vegetable

Cauliflower

> 1 small head fresh cauliflower
> Pam Cooking Spray

Soufflé

> 1/2 cup flour
> 2 cups skim or 1 percent low-fat milk
> 4 egg yolks
> 1/2 teaspoon Colman's dry mustard
> Small dash nutmeg and curry
> 7 egg whites
> 1 teaspoon salt
> 1/2 cup very finely grated Cheddar cheese

Remove cauliflower leaves and steam whole. Drain well. Spray a 3-quart soufflé dish with Pam. Place cauliflower in it.

To make soufflé, mix flour with small amount of milk to make a smooth paste. Add remaining milk gradually, to avoid lumps. Cook over low heat until smooth and thick, stirring constantly. Allow to cool and add egg yolks and seasonings. Mix well.

Allow egg whites to rest and come to room temperature. Beat them until very stiff; add salt and cheese to stiffly beaten whites and then fold into soufflé mixture. Pour over cauliflower. Bake in preheated 375°F oven, on center shelf, for about 40 to 45 minutes, or until well puffed and firm.

Serves 10 to 12 as a side dish.

Cost:	Moderate.
Calories:	105 per serving (based on 10 servings per recipe) (medium).

Preparation: Moderately difficult.
Comments: Crucifers and calcium *à la* Barbara Louria.

Apple–Sweet Potato Bake
Vegetable

3 large sweet potatoes, boiled until tender, skins removed
2 cooking apples, unpeeled but cored and sliced
1/3 cup yellow raisins
2 tablespoons brown sugar
1/4 cup coarsely chopped walnuts
1 teaspoon cinnamon
1/4 teaspoon ground nutmeg
2 tablespoons corn or safflower oil margarine
1/2 cup apple juice

Slice sweet potatoes crosswise into coin-shaped slices.
Arrange in a flat baking dish, alternating with apple slices,
and sprinkling each layer with raisins, brown sugar,
walnuts, cinnamon, and nutmeg. Dot with margarine and
pour apple juice over top. Cover and bake at 350°F for 40
minutes.

Serves 6.

Cost: Inexpensive.
Calories: 193 per serving (medium).
Preparation: Easy.
Comments: Great if you like sweet potatoes; provides plenty of carotenes and some fiber.

Minty Marinated Carrots   Vegetable

> 1 pound fresh carrots, peeled and cut into
>   julienne slices (cut in half lengthwise
>   and quarter each half)
> 1/2 cup red wine vinegar
> 1/4 cup olive oil
> 2 cloves fresh garlic, sliced thin
> 4 fresh mint leaves, chopped, or 1
>   teaspoon dried mint
> Salt to taste

Boil carrots in water to cover or steam in steamer basket for 15 minutes or until just tender, but not soft. Drain and cool. Mix vinegar, oil, garlic, mint, and salt. Marinate cooked carrots in this mixture overnight. Serve cold.

Serves 6.

Cost:	Inexpensive.
Calories:	110 per serving (medium).
Preparation:	Easy.
Comments:	Absolutely delicious and, of course, loaded with carotenes.

Frozen Yogurt Pops   Dessert

> 2 1/2 cups fresh or frozen strawberries,
>   raspberries, or blueberries (trimmed of
>   stems), or 2 ripe bananas
> 12 ounces vanilla low-fat yogurt
> 8 3- to 4-ounce paper cups
> 8 wooden sticks or plastic spoons

Place fruit and yogurt in blender. Cover and mix on medium speed until smooth and fruit is well blended. Fill paper cups and freeze for about 30 minutes until firm enough to hold a stick or plastic spoon in center of each cup. Freeze until solid. To serve, peel off paper.

Makes 8 pops.

Cost:	Inexpensive.
Calories:	50 to 100 (low).
Preparation:	Easy.
Comments:	Refreshing, particularly on a warm day. About 75 milligrams of calcium per pop.

Almond Custard with Fresh Fruit   Dessert

3/4 cup water
1/4 cup sugar
1 envelope unflavored gelatin
1 cup skim milk   •
1 teaspoon almond extract
Sliced fresh fruit such as: kiwi,
*   pineapple, strawberries, bananas, or*
*   mandarin orange sections*
Amaretto or other almond-flavored
*   liqueur (optional)*

Heat water, sugar, and gelatin to boiling, stirring occasionally until sugar and gelatin are dissolved. Remove from heat. Stir in milk and almond extract. Cover and refrigerate until firm, at least 4 hours. Cut gelatin custard into 1-inch diamonds or squares. Place several custard shapes into individual dessert dishes. Top with sliced fresh fruit and a teaspoon of almond liqueur.

Serves 4 to 6.

Cost:	Moderate.
Calories:	90 per serving (with Amaretto) (excluding fresh fruit) (low).
Preparation:	Moderately difficult.
Comments:	Offers a modicum of calcium, plus whatever advantages the individual fruits provide. Very low in fat.

7

Vitamins and
Aspirin

Our pharmaceutical cornucopia provides us with an extraordinary array of new substances every year, but today, in the forefront of current excitement, we can find two old, familiar groups—vitamins and aspirin.

Vitamins

There are three possible approaches to vitamin treatment. The first is to take vitamins containing the official recommended daily allowance (RDA)—the result of a consensus among nutrition experts and vitaminologists. These dosages change from time to time and represent little more than an educated guess, which does not adequately take into account the interactions among various constituents of the diet. Supposedly there is a built-in safety factor in the RDA levels, but that has not really been proved.

The second approach is to give two to three times the RDA —still considered a "conventional" dosage. This method has certain advantages, as it makes it more likely that adequate amounts of vitamins will reach the bloodstream and that patients of all ages will receive the correct amount.

The third approach is to take at least ten times the RDA of certain vitamins, the so-called megadoses. As yet, there is no evidence that megadoses of any vitamin will prevent disease in a normal, healthy person. There *are* cases of specific diseases in which megavitamins are helpful. For example, there is a very rare form of biotin deficiency in children that responds to massive biotin dosages. There is at present a great deal of enthusiasm for massive amounts of vitamins E and C, but neither, even in very large doses, will prevent heart attacks or cancer and neither prolongs the life of cancer victims, as some adherents think.

Some enthusiasts take massive doses of the B-complex vitamins—thiamin, niacin, riboflavin, and pyridoxine. None has been shown to be effective in preventing any disease. Vitamin A has been touted as an anticancer substance. In some experimental studies it is; in others, it is not. But vitamin A is stored in the liver and is not available to other tissues in large-enough amounts to be a cancer preventative. To get larger amounts to various tissues would require taking in so much vitamin A that vitamin A poisoning would result. Every one of the vitamins, if given in very large doses, can be the cause of illness that ranges in severity from mild to very severe, even fatal. Vitamins A and D, when given in large dosages, carry the greatest risk of severe adverse effects; there is no evidence that taking these very large doses confers any additional benefit. Megadoses carry a real risk of adverse side effects that on occasion can be life-threatening (see table 23).

Is the vitamin content of food such that a sensible, balanced diet provides all the vitamins needed? In January 1988, an expert panel of the American Institute of Nutrition and the American Society of Clinical Nutrition urged a balanced diet and advocated vitamin supplements only for pregnant women. They also advocated iron for menstruating women, and minerals plus B_{12} for vegetarians. In essence, they want to depend solely on the diet to get adequate vitamin intake. A similar recommendation was made by the National Research Council in March 1989 (see table 24).

It is difficult to understand the panel's overlooking the special needs of those over sixty years of age.

Fact: Most studies show that older persons frequently do not get even the RDAs in their diets. Older people often eat poorly for a lot of reasons—inadequate income, loss of taste and smell sensations (foods become less appetizing), loneliness, loss of interest in preparing adequate meals.

TABLE 23

Toxic Effects of Megadoses of Certain Vitamins and Excessive Amounts of Certain Minerals

Vitamin A	Skin abnormalities, hair loss, headache, blurred vision (even blindness), drowsiness, fatigue, bone damage, liver damage, possible fetal damage
Vitamin E	Fatigue, headache, increased cholesterol level, clots in veins, high blood pressure (these adverse effects occur uncommonly)
Vitamin C	Diarrhea, kidney stones (rare)
Pyridoxine (B$_6$)	Walking difficulties, sensory loss, limb impairment (may last for months after stopping pyridoxine)
Zinc	Nausea, vomiting, loss of appetite, lethargy, irritability, abdominal pain, anemia, fever, diarrhea, muscle pain
Selenium	Nausea, vomiting, loss of appetite, fatigue, skin discoloration, skin rash, dental caries, brittle nails, hair loss
Vitamin D	Headache, high blood pressure, nausea, weakness, vomiting, diarrhea, kidney failure, bone pain

---

Fact: Some older people may not absorb certain vitamins adequately. For example, they may not absorb the more complex forms of folic acid in foods, but they *can* absorb the simpler forms of folic acid in vitamin pills.

TABLE 24

Vitamin Availability in Foods

Several portions of servings each week in each category will provide adequate vitamins for most people.

Vitamin	Major Sources
A	Milk; liver; spinach; fish liver oils; carrots; green and yellow fruits and vegetables; egg yolk
B_1 (thiamin)	Meats; poultry; peanuts; brown rice; fish; molasses; oatmeal; wheat germ; green peas; dried beans
B_2 (riboflavin)	Whole wheat, rye, or pumpernickel breads; liver; kidneys; sweetbreads; molasses; Brussels sprouts; milk, cheese, yogurt; broccoli; beet greens; asparagus; bean sprouts
B_6 (pyridoxine)	Various meats; liver; kidneys; sweetbreads; whole wheat, rye, or pumpernickel breads; brown rice; peas; navy beans; molasses; green leafy vegetables; fish; poultry; potato; beef liver; banana
B_{12}	Meats; cheese; fish; milk; liver; kidneys; tuna fish; eggs
Biotin	Peas; beans; whole wheat, rye, or pumpernickel breads; lentils; eggs; liver; soybeans
Folic acid	Milk; green leafy vegetables; oysters; salmon; tuna fish; whole wheat, rye, or pumpernickel breads; spinach; dates
Niacin	Meats; seafoods; milk; poultry; peanuts; liver; rhubarb
Pantothenic acid	Peas; beans; orange juice; liver; salmon; mushrooms; whole wheat, rye, or pumpernickel breads
C (ascorbic acid)	Citrus fruits; strawberries; broccoli; green peppers; cantaloupe; tomatoes
D	Egg yolk; liver; kidneys; milk; salmon; tuna fish; sweetbreads; cereals (only those cereals fortified with vitamin D)
E	Green vegetables; eggs; liver; kidneys; sweetbreads; oatmeal; vegetable oils (soybean, cottonseed, corn, safflower), wheat germ

NOTE: The foods listed are particularly plentiful in the vitamin indicated, but there are many other foods containing these vitamins; some foods also have vitamins added by the manufacturers. Ideally, vegetables are eaten raw or cooked quickly without water. The longer the cooking in water, the greater the likelihood of loss of vitamins.

Fact: Older people often have striking deficiencies in blood levels of many vitamins. The only ones who predictably have adequate levels are those taking vitamin supplements.

Fact: There are interactions among constituents of the diet and some of the interactions will reduce vitamin absorption from the intestines into the bloodstream. There are many such interactions, many of which are poorly understood. It is possible that the many of the prescription and over-the-counter medications that older persons take may have negative effects on vitamin absorption.

In my judgment, it is a mistake simply to tell people over sixty to eat well. Too many of them will end up vitamin-deficient.

What will a vitamin supplement do for older persons? It will assure them of adequate levels of vitamins in the blood. For those who are vitamin-deficient, and perhaps even for those whose blood vitamin levels appear normal, the vitamin supplement may give them more energy and vitality. There are no guarantees of this, but certainly for those over age sixty who feel washed out or listless, a vitamin supplement is advisable (see table 25).

There is some new information in one area that is very exciting. Dr. John Bogden of the New Jersey Medical School was studying the effect of zinc on immunity in older persons; such persons often have immunologic defects that favor certain infections and may increase susceptibility to some cancers. In very meticulous studies, he found no effect of zinc, but each group, including those given two different doses of zinc and the controls given no zinc, showed rather striking improvement in immunity. This surprising finding could possibly have been due to the way the study was carried out, but it is much more likely that improved immunity was related to the supplemental vitamins given to all groups to make sure the groups were comparable.

Obviously, these findings need to be confirmed and Dr. Bogden must make sure it was indeed the standard vitamin supplement that improved immunity. But the implications and potential of that study are mind-boggling. One of the

TABLE 25

Tips for Those Taking Vitamins, Calcium, or Iron

Advice	Reason
Take multivitamin supplements with or after meals.	Often better absorption.
Do not consume carbonated soda drinks two hours before or two hours after taking calcium tablets.	Soft drinks have high content of phosphates, which will reduce calcium absorption.
Vitamin supplements should not be taken within four hours of taking sodium bicarbonate or other antacids.	Riboflavin and thiamin are destroyed by these alkaline substances.
Antacids should not be taken within four hours of taking multivitamins.	Acid in the stomach is needed for vitamin C absorption.
If you are taking tetracycline drugs, wait at least two hours before taking vitamins.	Tetracyclines can interfere with absorption.
Orange juice, if taken about the same time as iron, will increase iron absorption.	Vitamin C will increase iron absorption.
Don't use milk to wash down vitamin capsules or tablets.	The milk will interfere with absorption of some vitamins.
If you use mineral oil regularly as a laxative, vitamins A and D (and perhaps K) may be absorbed less.	The mineral oil acts on the intestines to reduce absorption of these vitamins.
If you are taking anticoagulant drugs, do not take large doses of vitamin E.	The large doses of vitamin E can increase the tendency to experience bleeding from the anticoagulants.

most important deficits affecting many older people is impairment of the immune system. Deterioration in the immune system has been related not only to increased susceptibility to certain infections and cancers, but also to reduction in life expectancy. If conventional doses of vitamins can help the immune system stay young as we get older, and thus increase resistance to some infections and to some cancers, and perhaps even prolong life, that would be extraordinary. There would then be additional support for the recommendation that every person sixty years of age or older take a conventional dose of a vitamin supplement every day. It might even be prudent to lower to fifty the age for starting supplemental vitamins as a preventive measure for maintaining immunity. A derivative question would then be, "Which vitamins are the ones responsible for the improvement in immunity?" That will take years of research to answer, and it may not be a single vitamin. It might be that one vitamin is effective for some people, another for another group of aging persons; or it might be that two or more vitamins acting in concert is what is required. A report by Dr. Simin Nikbin Meydani of the Human Nutrition Research Center on Aging at Tufts University in Boston in 1989 suggested that vitamin E might be important for older persons. She noted improvement in immune responses in seventeen elderly persons after one month of vitamin E supplementation.

We still have too many gaps in our knowledge and there is too much hyperbole and hogwash foisted on the public about taking vitamins. But these recent studies are enormously interesting. Vitamins represent long-known chemicals that may be extremely useful when taken in moderation and for appropriate, documented purposes.

Can taking vitamins in conventional (or megadoses) help prevent cancer? There are now at least a dozen studies on vitamin E. About half say there is at least some protection against certain cancers; the other half find no protection at all. The best summary statement at present is that there is no persuasive evidence that vitamin E or any other vitamin taken in any dose protects an individual from the development of any cancer.

Will vitamin supplements improve or sustain memory and intellectual vigor? Nobody knows. Surprisingly, this has never been adequately tested. We appear to have accepted the notion that older persons should expect to lose intellectual zest and forget things. That makes little sense. Memory loss is due to changes in the physiology and biochemistry of the brain. For most people, it should not be inevitable. Very few people would have thought it possible that simple vitamin supplementation could reverse the immunity deficits that affect many older persons; but that may indeed be the case. The situation with thinking and memory could be similar. Only now are some of the skeptics beginning to acknowledge that vitamin supplements could improve thinking, memory, feelings of well-being, and the quality of life.

Will taking vitamins improve sexuality or sexual potency for older persons? There is no evidence that it will, but like intellectual functioning, it has not been adequately studied. Here, again, nobody knows. But loss of sexual vigor should not have to be inevitable and should be at least partially avoidable. If vitamins can modify immunity, they could also improve feelings of well-being, sexuality being a part of that.

The role of vitamins in improving feelings of general well-being, memory, intellectual vigor, sexuality is not established, but we do not need to wait for proof in these areas to make some sensible recommendations. Those over age sixty should be taking a vitamin supplement, anyway, and if vitamins can be shown to improve immunity (as they may well do), then probably everyone over age fifty should be taking a vitamin supplement. If that vitamin supplement also improves memory, vigor, thinking, the quality of life, or sexuality, in any combination, so much the better.

I used to feel that a good diet was all that was needed and that only pregnant women needed a vitamin supplement. I have modified that view because older people may not absorb some vitamins as well from the intestinal tract and because the multiple prescription and nonprescription drugs taken by older people may reduce the availability or absorption of vitamins in the foods they eat. And of course the possibility that vitamins may help keep the immune system young is very exciting.

What kind of vitamin supplement do I recommend? Herman Baker, Ph.D., an expert on vitamins, and John Bogden, Ph.D., an expert on trace nutrients, and I examined available vitamin preparations and found none entirely satisfactory. To overcome the reduced absorption in some older persons and the potential reduction in vitamin availability because of prescription or nonprescription drugs, we decided to formulate a new vitamin preparation, containing for the most part about three times the RDA and including only those vitamins and trace nutrients for which we believe there is reasonable evidence supporting their inclusion. That formulation is given in table 26. It will be manufactured and distributed by Schiff Products, Inc., a leading distributor of vitamins, and will be called "Vita 3." We believe that 0.8 milligrams is most desirable for folic acid, but the FDA does not permit more than 0.4 milligrams in over-the-counter supplements. Schiff also produces a tablet with 0.4 milligrams of folic acid. I advocate one of these along with one a day of Vita 3.

Although this is formulated specifically for those over age sixty, it is actually a good formulation for any adult who takes vitamins.

Aspirin

It is said that aspirin will prevent a heart attack or stroke, or will prevent a second heart attack after one has already occurred, or will prevent stroke after premonitory signs of stroke are present. All this is based on its anticlotting properties. Millions of people are taking aspirin as a preventative. Some take one a day, others two a day, and still others three to four or more a day.

Aspirin has *not* been shown convincingly to prevent heart attacks in apparently healthy people. Only two studies have been performed, with completely different results. One study was carried out in the United States, one in England; both were published in January 1988. One showed a marked reduction in heart attack risk by taking small amounts of aspirin, but the other study showed no protection at all and both

TABLE 26

Vita 3 Formulation
(recommended dosage—one a day)

Vitamin A	5,000 IU*
Vitamin E	50 IU
Vitamin C	200 milligrams
Vitamin B_1	4 milligrams
Vitamin B_2	5 milligrams
Niacin	50 milligrams
Vitamin B_6	7 milligrams
Pantothenic acid	25 milligrams
Biotin	500 micrograms
Folic acid	0.4 (0.8) milligrams[†]
Vitamin B_{12}	30 micrograms
Iron	10 milligrams
Vitamin D	400 IU
Selenium	50 micrograms
Chromium	0.1 milligrams
Beta carotene	30 milligrams

*IU = international units.

[†]The FDA does not permit more than 0.4 milligrams of folic acid in nonprescription vitamins; to get 0.8 milligrams a day will require an additional folic acid tablet.

studies found a small increase in the risk of disabling strokes among aspirin-takers. Since the two studies, both carried out by excellent investigators, are so divergent, no conclusion and no recommendation is possible.

What about secondary prevention? That is, administering aspirin to those who have had a heart attack or a stroke or a severe form of angina (heart-related chest pain) or a transient ischemic attack (in essence, a brief, mild stroke that can lead to a full-blown stroke)? The evidence here is a lot more persuasive. In the January 30, 1988, issue of the *British Medical Journal,* a total of twenty aspirin studies were carefully analyzed. Although some of the studies were negative, most showed encouraging results. For all studies combined, those taking aspirin, compared with controls not given aspirin, showed a one-third decrease in the likelihood of subsequent nonfatal heart attack or stroke and a 15 percent reduction in risk of developing a fatal stroke or heart attack.

One aspirin tablet a day was just as effective as four aspirin tablets a day. There is a strong likelihood that for some people, the aspirin is disadvantageous, producing bleeding into the head and perhaps disabling or fatal strokes, but this is outweighed by the beneficial effects. Still, candidates for aspirin must be chosen carefully. Only those with a documented stroke, transient ischemic attack, heart attack, or angina are candidates on the basis of current evidence.

What about aspirin as treatment *after* a heart attack has occurred? The data here are very exciting. There are now two studies that have quite similar conclusions. If a patient has a heart attack and is given an aspirin tablet a day for up to a month, plus one injection of a substance called streptokinase to dissolve blood clots in the heart, and if the aspirin is started within twenty-four hours of the onset of the heart attack (preferably within four hours), there is a 40 to 50 percent reduction in deaths as a result of the heart attack. If aspirin is given alone (without the streptokinase or a similar clot-dissolving drug), there is a 20 to 25 percent reduction in deaths. That is impressive. It is true that more studies are needed, but the data currently available look very good.

Some researchers now say that if you have severe chest pain and are convinced you are having a heart attack, it would make sense to take an aspirin tablet as you go to the doctor's office or, more likely, to the hospital. Taking one aspirin tablet (no more) is probably a good idea under those circumstances, but only if you are going to see a doctor shortly.

In summary, aspirin has not been shown persuasively to

prevent heart attacks or strokes in healthy people. Aspirin given daily in small amounts does appear useful in preventing strokes or heart attacks in those who have already had a stroke, a heart attack, recurrent heart pain (angina) or a minor stroke. Aspirin seems to be helpful, taken promptly and in small dosage, in reducing the likelihood of death after a heart attack (as part of comprehensive treatment for that heart attack). Like vitamins, aspirin is an ancient substance that, when used correctly, has remarkable benefits.

8

Additional
Thoughts

The goal of the Health-Full-Life Program is to provide the maximum benefit for a minimum expenditure of time and money. We want you to take charge of your own health. To accomplish that goal, we try to be careful about adding inadequately documented recommendations to our program. This would be a disservice, and inevitably reduce the benefit to the public.

There are literally hundreds of new recommendations every year: saccharin is a dangerous drug; coffee drinking is related to cancer of the pancreas or bowel; changes must be made in the Type A personality to reduce heart attack risk; fat in the diet causes breast cancer; and on and on.

None of these assertions is documented; the relationship between coffee drinking and pancreatic cancer is a typical example of the history of many such claims. In 1981, with great fanfare, the *New England Journal of Medicine* published an article originating at the Harvard School of Public Health showing that coffee drinking appeared to be a risk factor for cancer of the pancreas, a cancer whose occurrence means almost certain death in a few months for the victim. The chief author of that study, an eminent epidemiologist, reported on television that one study did not prove that coffee drinking played a role in pancreatic cancer, but the results would certainly influence him to reduce coffee drinking, or perhaps to stop it altogether. The public was properly scared. But, in fact, it was not a very good study, it did not merit publication in the *New England Journal of Medicine,* and when all the hullabaloo died down, several studies showing no such association were reported.

Unfortunately, negative studies usually do not get a great deal of public attention. Five years later, in the August 28, 1986, issue of the *New England Journal of Medicine,* a brief letter appeared entitled, "Coffee and Pancreatic Cancer (Chapter 2)." It was again from the Harvard School of Public Health, written by the same authors (with one addition). They had redone the study. This time, no such association was found. In a paradigm of understatement, they concluded that "if there is any association between coffee consumption and cancer of the pancreas, it is not as strong as our earlier data suggested." It sure isn't. As a matter of fact, the association doesn't exist at all.

In general, in the area of health, we should do what is supported by adequate evidence, and keep the costs down. Even then, some experts will assert programs such as Health-Full-Life are not cost-effective. Our own analysis of the total Health-Full-Life Program, performed by a statistician not connected with the program, indicates it *is* cost-effective, saving an employer at least two dollars for every dollar spent; but all such calculations are open to debate because each is based on a variety of assumptions, and different experts use different assumptions. If prevention is not cost-effective, if it does not actually save money, then the question is, how much are we willing to spend to maximize the chances of staying healthy and thus improve the quality and duration of life? In any case, keeping the costs as low as possible is highly desirable.

Alcohol

I have said little about alcohol. That is because I have little to say that is helpful. Moderation is the key word. One or two alcoholic drinks a day may actually be good for the heart; moderate alcohol intake appears to offer some protection against heart attacks and apparently does so by raising HDL levels. But as many as one-third of those who drink one or two drinks a day will at some time have a drinking problem that may far outweigh any benefits that one or two drinks a day can confer on the heart.

If you drink alcohol, do so in moderation, advice that is hardly apocalyptic, but there are potential dangers. For instance, people who have two drinks and then drive are sometimes in automobile accidents, and it seems clear that for pregnant women, one glass of wine a day, or its equivalent, should be the maximum. Alcohol in excess is a risk factor for esophagus and larynx cancer, as well as the major cause of liver cirrhosis, one of the leading causes of death in the United States. And the association of alcohol intake and breast cancer is still unsettled; the evidence is suggestive, but certainly not proven. In May 1987, two articles in the *New England Journal of Medicine* about alcohol and breast cancer produced headlines in newspapers across the country. The first article was by Arthur Schatzkin, M.D., and multiple co-authors from the National Cancer Institute in Bethesda, Maryland; the second was by Walter C. Willett, M.D., and his colleagues from the Harvard Medical School.

The investigators from the National Cancer Institute questioned 7,188 women, twenty-five to seventy-four years of age, considered to be a representative sample of the U.S. population. They were followed for a period that ranged from six to thirteen years, during which time 121 cases of breast cancer occurred. The researchers found that any drinking of alcohol, even of a very small amount, increased the risk by about 50 percent, but there was no dose-response relationship—that is, heavier drinkers did not have an appreciably greater risk than very modest or even very light users of alcohol. The increased risk was noted even among women who consumed fewer than three drinks a week, a very small amount. The risk appeared greater for younger, premenopausal women.

The Harvard study is larger; almost 90,000 registered nurses were enrolled in 1980; during the next four years, 601 cases of breast cancer were diagnosed. For those women who consumed three to nine drinks a week, there was a 30 percent increased risk of breast cancer. Those who drank more than one drink a day had a 50 percent increase in breast cancer risk. The authors concluded "Our findings in conjunction with those of previous studies indicate that an association exists that is unlikely to be the result of chance."

These are solid studies. Previously, there had been multiple case-control studies in which a case of known breast cancer was matched with a control. About two-thirds of those studies showed alcohol to be a risk factor, but one-third did not. Additionally, there were considerable problems with methodology among the positive studies, and there were many discrepant results. There are now three prospective studies (including these two) in which women were selected who did not have breast cancer and were followed for a number of years to study the subsequent occurrence of the disease. All three studies found a relationship, but there were differences: one found *any* drinking put the patient at risk; one found a few drinks a week resulted in increased risk; and one study found that only those who drank three alcoholic drinks a day were at increased risk.

The extent of the increased risk was moderate, but still significant. It is a bit bothersome that the dose-response effect was not striking; one would have expected a more impressive gradient in risks as the daily (or weekly) alcohol dosage increased.

It is hard to make a public health recommendation until more is known about the dividing line between the amount of alcohol that produces minimal (if any) increase in risk of developing breast cancer, and the amount of alcohol that definitely increases the risk.

Before going overboard, it should be noted that at the Society for Epidemiologic Research meetings in June 1987 and June 1988, there were two reasonably good studies showing no relationship between alcohol consumption and breast cancer. Furthermore, in the May 20, 1988, issue of the *Journal of the American Medical Association,* Randall E. Harris, Ph.D., and Ernst Wynder, M.D., one of our best epidemiologists, reported a study of 1,467 breast cancer cases. They found no evidence of any association between alcohol intake and breast cancer. They point out that if alcohol plays any role, it is a very weak one. I believe that until someone shows a *strong* association between alcohol consumption and breast cancer, we should just forget the issue.

Coffee

I have not said anything about coffee. It is well known that very heavy coffee drinking can be associated with heart rhythm irregularities; and women with nontumorous lumps in the breast (so-called fibrocystic disease) are advised to reduce their coffee intake. Some studies have linked heavy coffee consumption with cancers other than pancreas cancer, but none of these investigations has been persuasive. Heavy coffee intake has also been linked to heart attacks. The best of these studies was published in the October 16, 1986, *New England Journal of Medicine.* Andrea Z. LaCroix and her colleagues from the Johns Hopkins Medical Institutions in Baltimore, Maryland, followed 1,130 men for nineteen to thirty-five years and found that the risk for those drinking five cups a day was more than twice the risk for nonusers. However, many other studies are negative and, at present, pending additional studies, coffee drinking cannot be directly associated either with heart attacks or cancer. The prudent recommendation about coffee, like alcohol, is moderation. I personally feel the definition of moderation for most people is no more than three to five cups a day (two to three cups for a pregnant woman) but some of my colleagues would recommend a maximum of three cups a day.

Oral Contraceptives

Women on the pill get clots in the legs, heart attacks, and strokes more frequently than women of the same age not taking oral contraceptives. Fortunately, such heart attacks and strokes occur rarely. Furthermore, those who do have heart attacks usually have other risk factors, including diabetes, high blood pressure, elevated cholesterol, or low levels of high-density lipoproteins. They are also likely to be heavy smokers—over a pack a day.

Any woman taking oral contraceptives should be examined for risk factors; if she has hypertension, diabetes, elevated cholesterol, or low levels of high-density lipoproteins, she should use alternate methods of contraception. And, if a woman does take oral contraceptives, she should certainly not smoke more than half a pack of cigarettes per day.

Oral contraceptives appear to reduce the chances of getting uterine or ovarian cancer. The evidence for this is quite persuasive. On the negative side, young women taking the pill may increase their risk of developing breast cancer, and those using oral contraceptives for more than ten years may have some increased risk of developing cervical cancer. So oral contraceptive pills definitely reduce the risk of two female cancers and may increase the risk of two others. If all the cancers are considered together, oral contraceptives actually reduce the cancer risk somewhat.

Recently there has been a flurry of increased concern about the influence of the pill on breast cancer because of three studies—one from Boston, published in the *American Journal of Epidemiology* in February 1989, one from England, and one from the Centers for Disease Control in Atlanta.

The studies actually came to different conclusions and all applied only to women less than forty-five years of age. Only a small percentage of breast cancers affect young women, age forty-five or less.

The Boston study concluded that any use of oral contraceptives doubled the risk of breast cancer occurring before age forty-five.

The British study said that there is increased risk among takers of the pill, but only if the woman had one child.

The Centers for Disease Control study suggested an increased risk, but only for women who had no children and started menstruating before age thirteen.

The authors of the Boston study spent most of the discussion part of their report saying they cannot explain their findings and that they themselves in a prior study found no such association between oral contraceptives and breast cancer; one author of the Centers for Disease Control study is quoted as saying that oral contraceptives have no significant impact on breast cancer.

Thus, the studies are not convergent and the authors are not certain of their own findings. That being the case, the public should not take the results too seriously.

Diet and Cancer Prevention

I have repeatedly talked about diet and health because it is an important topic and one that is much on the minds of the public. One question often asked is What should you do with regard to diet to prevent cancer?

It is now the fad to say that a lot of cancer is dietary in origin and, therefore, can be prevented by diet. Table 27 summarizes the reports of publications that apportion the risk factors for cancer occurrence. The largest single risk factor is said to be the diet, more important than smoking, a fully documented cause of cancer. But the 35 percent ascribed to diet is all supposition; in actuality, the percentage may be a lot less. At present, the assumption that dietary intake relates to a significant percentage of cancers is an interesting notion that is not adequately documented.

The relationship of animal protein intake to cancer is inadequately documented either in man or experimental animals, but the relationship between animal fat and cancer is somewhat more impressive. There are many experiments in which the animals (usually rats) have been given a substance to cause tumors and then given supplementary fats in the diet. In those fat-supplemented animals, the tumor incidence is increased substantially; both saturated and polyunsaturated fats appear to promote such cancers.

Many substances given to rats or other laboratory animals promote cancers, and it is dangerous to apply rat results to the human condition. The two cancers thought to be most directly linked to fat intake involve the bowel and breast. A 1989 study from the Harvard School of Public Health indi-

TABLE 27

Alleged Causes of Cancer

Cause	Percent
Diet	35
Tobacco	30
Occupation	4
Alcohol	3
Viruses	5
Environmental pollution	2
Sunshine	3

cated that greater animal fat consumption increased the risk of colon cancer about twofold; the animal fat consumed was mainly beef. However, people in Finland take in a great deal of animal fat, but have relatively low bowel cancer rates. Seventh-Day Adventists are frequently vegetarian and they have low bowel cancer rates. This has been ascribed to their low intake of animal fat, but Mormons have the same reduction in bowel cancer incidence, yet have an animal fat intake similar to the average American. At present, the notion that reducing fat intake will lower the risk of bowel cancer is not adequately documented.

What about breast cancer? The recommendations for lowering fat intake from the present more than 40 percent to less than 30 percent as a method of reducing the risk of breast cancer by 35 to 50 percent is based on four observations: international studies show a much lower risk of breast cancer in countries that consume lower amounts of fat; those migrating from countries with low breast cancer rates to countries with high breast cancer rates tend to increase their rate of breast cancer; animals given a chemical to cause breast cancer show more cancers if given a diet higher in saturated or unsaturated fats; some studies comparing breast cancer cases and controls show that those with breast cancer had more fat in their diets.

Walter C. Willett, M.D., and his colleagues reported in the January 1, 1987, *New England Journal of Medicine* that a study of almost 90,000 nurses showed no correlation at all between fat intake and breast cancer. One negative study is not conclusive, but the Willett study is the best carried out to date, and it strongly implies that our present national guidelines in regard to fat intake and breast cancer prevention should not be taken too seriously until more data are available. Two studies in 1988 on Seventh-Day Adventists by a well-known group at Loma Linda University gave no comfort to those who support the notion of a link between animal fat intake and breast cancer. Seventh-Day Adventists include total vegetarians, vegetarians who also include dairy products and eggs in their diet, and meat eaters. The risk of breast cancer was the same in all three groups. On the other hand, a study of 250 breast cancer cases in Italy published February 15, 1989, in the *Journal of the National Cancer Institute,* concluded that saturated fat in dairy products (as well as a high intake of calories and animal protein) significantly increases the risk of breast cancer. So the jury is still out in regard to fat intake and breast cancer.

It seems unlikely that reduction in dietary fat to a modest extent (from 40 percent of total calories to 30 percent) will reduce the risk of breast cancer. Perhaps if the fat intake is lowered to 20 percent or less, the breast cancer risk would fall, but that would require a very restrictive diet; it is unlikely that many women would follow such a diet.

Now that an adequate period of time has passed to permit careful analysis of the concept that a high-fiber diet is a protector against bowel cancer, there are questions. Currently, its relationship can only be listed as an uncertain possibility. To me, the current situation can be summarized as follows:

- The majority of the data support eating a reasonable amount of fiber (20 to 30 grams in an adult); this is likely to help in preventing certain inflammatory diseases of the bowel, including diverticulitis and appendicitis.
- Excessive fiber intake might be harmful.
- We still have a great deal to learn about the role of various types of fiber.
- It is improper to make ill-documented claims about cancer prevention. Some of the alleged protection against colon-rectal cancer could be due not to the fiber, but to other constituents of vegetables that are also high in fiber content.
- It might well be that some types of fiber are beneficial and other types are ineffective or actually harmful.

There is increasing interest not only in fiber types (soluble versus insoluble), but also in the source of the fiber. For example, an interesting study by J. L. Freudenheim and her colleagues from State University of New York at Buffalo concerning dietary fiber and rectal cancer was presented at the June 1989 meeting of the Society for Epidemiologic Research.

They studied 422 rectal cancer cases and an equal number of controls. Intake of soluble and insoluble fiber in fruits and vegetables appeared to be protective against rectal cancer, reducing the risk by about half. In contrast, eating a lot of soluble and insoluble grain fiber had no protective effect at all. In other words, fiber in grains is different from fiber in fruits and vegetables. All those advertisements about eating a lot of cereal grains to prevent bowel cancer may be incorrect. There are now several studies suggesting (but not yet proving) that as far as bowel cancer is concerned, eating ample quantities of fiber-containing fruits and vegetables may be much more desirable than eating all those cereals. If certain fruits and vegetables are protective, it may not be their fiber content; they also contain, for example, substantial amounts of carotenes that could be protective.

Fruits and vegetables that contain at least three grams of

dietary fiber per serving include: apple, banana, blueberries (one cup), dates (ten), figs (ten), nectarine, orange, papaya, pear, dried prunes (ten), raspberries (one cup), rhubarb (one-half cup), strawberries (one cup), broccoli, spinach, sweet potato, corn, lima beans, peas, baked beans, kidney beans, lentils, black-eyed peas, and split peas.

In late 1983 and early 1984, the National Cancer Institute, the National Academy of Sciences, and the American Cancer Society all advocated an anticancer diet of less fat, more fiber, less salt-cured or smoked meat, increased intake of cruciferous vegetables, and more vitamin C and carotene-containing foods. Although they promoted this as an anticancer diet, they were reasonably cautious, but some of my colleagues who were quoted were not, and suggested that this diet would prevent 75 percent of colon cancers, 50 percent of breast cancers, and up to 50 percent of prostate cancers. These glib pronouncements are unabashed hyperbole. There is no diet that will assure you that you will be less likely to get cancer. The recommended diet does make sense. It is good for the heart, and *might* be helpful in preventing cancer, but that is as far as we can go. To say it will definitely prevent one-third to three-quarters of cancers of the colon, breast, and prostate is pure hogwash.

Dietary Supplements

Zinc is supposed to restore taste and smell sensations in older people, but the evidence is so poor that zinc supplements cannot be recommended for that purpose. It may be that zinc will be found helpful in older persons, who often show age-related deficiencies in their immune system. In preliminary studies, the immune defects were partially reversed by administering zinc-containing capsules, but a more sophisticated and meticulous study by John Bogden, Ph.D., of the New Jersey Medical School found no evidence that zinc administration reversed the immune defects found in older people. Nevertheless, it does make sense to get adequate amounts of zinc in the diet; dark poultry meat, oysters, crab, veal, liver, and beef are major sources.

Selenium is like vitamin E in some respects. In experimental animals, it does indeed retard tumor growth. Does it have an antitumor effect in humans? Some say it does, but nobody really knows, and there is not much leeway between a potentially effective concentration of selenium and the toxic range. And we do not know nearly enough about the toxic effects of too much selenium, including the possibility that at high concentrations selenium could *promote* some tumors. The March 30, 1984, issue of *Morbidity and Mortality* told of a fifty-seven-year-old woman who took selenium in excessive dosage and developed nausea, vomiting, total baldness, swelling of her fingers, a sour odor to her breath, and abnormalities of her nails. Anyone taking selenium should be very careful not to exceed 100 to 200 micrograms daily.

Lecithin is said to be effective in large doses in lowering cholesterol levels and improving memory. There is no credible evidence it lowers cholesterol. It is true that several reports suggest that lecithin can improve memory defects in persons with certain severe disease, but most studies are negative and a careful review in 1980 in the British journal *Lancet* was not encouraging. At present, there is no justification for taking large amounts of lecithin.

Cholesterol-Lowering Drugs

Until relatively recently, no reasonably safe drug was available for general use that would lower blood cholesterol levels and/or raise high-density protein (HDL) levels. Now there are five and more are on the way. The most interesting is called lovastatin, which interferes with the body's manufacture of cholesterol. Only a small number of persons have been treated, but, in those, cholesterol levels fell as much as 40 percent, and HDL rose significantly. Another drug, called colestipol, works by increasing cholesterol excretion in the intestinal tract; so does another drug, cholestyramine. The fourth is niacin, the vitamin, and nobody is quite sure how it works. Then there is gemfibrozil. Gemfibrozil is a new drug that also lowers cholesterol and strikingly increases protective HDL levels. Studies in Finland show that administration of the drug to middle-aged men reduces the likelihood of subsequent heart attack. It is indeed encouraging that these drugs are available, and that exciting new ones are being developed, but everyone should remember that with drugs there are no guaranteed free rides. Niacin in the dosage used produces unpleasant flushes and hot, burning sensations that cause many people to refuse to take it. Colestipol tastes like gritty sand, causes constipation and sometimes very unpleasant feelings of fullness and bloating of the abdomen. Lovastatin can produce abnormalities of liver function, cataracts, and perhaps very annoying sleep disorders, as well as muscle inflammation. Approximately 10 percent of those given lovastatin show significant side effects. More than 10 percent of those given gemfibrozil have substantial abdominal complaints, and there are concerns about gallstones and eye cataracts.

That is why prudent doctors insist that for most people with mild to moderate elevations of cholesterol, weight loss, often together with physical exercise (to help with weight control), and a low-fat diet is the best and safest way to reduce cholesterol levels and hopefully to raise HDL levels. Drug use should be reserved for those with very high levels of cholesterol in the blood or inability to lower cholesterol or raise HDL after reasonably long and conscientious efforts without drugs. Reasonably long, to me, ordinarily means at least a year. In most cases, willpower and persistence as well as experimentation with different food patterns and exercises will be effective. Those who turn to drugs after a limited, desultory attempt at weight loss, exercise, and dietary modification put themselves at risk of adverse reactions to the drugs, and some undesirable side reactions may not become fully documented and well known for many years, even decades.

Interestingly, an article in the June 16, 1989, *Journal of the American Medical Association* indicated that the laxative

Metamucil, which is composed primarily of soluble fiber, lowered the blood cholesterol to a moderate degree when given in dosages of one teaspoon three times a day. Although interesting, these findings are preliminary; we need more studies and more information on whether the beneficial effects are sustained over periods of several months or years.

Coronary heart disease is the leading cause of death in the United States. The two major events that result from arteriosclerosis and subsequent narrowing of the coronary blood vessels of the heart are heart attacks (myocardial infarcts) and sudden death. Each year in the United States there are some 540,000 heart attacks that end fatally, including 250,000 cases of sudden death due to coronary heart disease. There are three approaches to reducing this scourge. One is to treat heart attacks more effectively. That is surely responsible for some of the remarkable 30 percent drop in heart disease deaths in the United States in the last two decades. A second approach is to treat more effectively those who have early symptoms of coronary heart disease (such as chest pains after exercise). We surely are doing that both with better medicines and with surgery on the coronary blood vessels if they can be shown to have severe narrowing from arteriosclerosis. The third approach, the best from the point of view of those in preventive medicine, is to find those who have important risk factors that promote coronary heart disease (high blood pressure, smoking, high cholesterol levels) and improve those risk factors.

There is an additional consideration. Perhaps 20 to 25 percent of all heart attacks are unrecognized (discovered only later by routine cardiograms in doctors' offices). The pressing question is how to recognize these persons before the heart attacks occur, as well as the estimated fifty thousand cases of sudden death each year who never had previous symptoms and the thousands more each year whose first evidence of heart disease is a fatal heart attack. There are now a growing number of cardiologists who believe that this can be done. It seems that perhaps 1 million to 2 million men age thirty-five to sixty years have a disease called silent myocardial ischemia. These are episodes of reduced blood supply to the heart muscle detected only by careful monitoring of the heart by a continuous electrocardiogram (a Holter monitor) or by changes on the cardiogram during an exercise test on a treadmill (a stress test). Supposedly, the evidence shows that persons with no symptoms who have significant, severe, or prolonged abnormalities on the Holter twenty-four-hour monitor or on the exercise stress test have a much greater chance of developing heart attacks or sudden death. The evidence, summarized in a recent book entitled *Silent Myocardial Ischemia and Angina,* edited by Bramah N. Singh, M.D. (Permagon Press, 1988), is thought by many to be so convincing that they feel that at-risk men should undergo an exercise stress test or have a Holter monitor. If specific changes are found in these electrocardiograms, they should have further tests and then coronary catheterization with angiography (a picture of the coronary vessels after injection of a dye). If severe narrowing is found, then the vessels can be dilated or coronary artery surgery can be performed.

A derivative question is, then, who should be tested? In a recent court decision, an award of $500,000 was made in the case of a man in his forties who had a family history of heart disease, had high blood pressure and an elevated cholesterol level, and smoked heavily. He died suddenly from coronary artery disease. The lawyers argued that the man was at high risk for coronary heart disease and heart attack and that a stress test should have been carried out even though he had no symptoms.

There are a welter of issues:

1. The stress test and the twenty-four-hour Holter monitoring produce a lot of false positive results—persons who test positive but after extensive subsequent testing are found to have no significant coronary artery disease. These are thought to be the 1 million to 2 million men with silent ischemia, but there are about 25 million men in that age group, so only about 5 to 10 percent of men this age have the disease in question. Most of the posi-

tive tests will be false positives; the likelihood of an apparently positive test being a true positive is only 25 to 35 percent.

2. The follow-up of a positive stress test or Holter monitor includes the injection of dyes to visualize the coronary blood vessels; this occasionally can cause severe allergic reactions (even death). So, the work-up is not totally without dangers—and the majority of persons will turn out not to have a serious disease.

3. The cost of all this work-up is very expensive—about $200 to $300 for a stress test, $150 to $250 for a Holter monitor. If these tests are positive, the additional study of the coronary blood vessels will cost at least $1,000 to $2,000. And in most cases they will not find serious coronary artery disease that needs immediate intervention.

4. It is not clear who should be screened. To reduce costs, and the dangers and costs inherent in working up false positives, it has been suggested that a man over age forty should be screened if he has, in addition to his age and sex, another risk factor, including a high cholesterol, high blood pressure, or a family history of heart attacks at an early age in a close relative. But the definition of a high cholesterol is changing. If the new "ideal" level of 200 or less is used for the cholesterol cut-off, we will be screening almost everyone—some say that is what the cardiologists really want.

   Some doctors will want to include as risk factors Type A personalities, others borderline hypertension. At present, there are no precise or consistent guidelines about who should be tested; and that is a real problem.

5. There is no consensus about the frequency of stress test or Holter monitor screening for those allegedly at high risk. Coronary artery disease is not static; cholesterol gets into blood vessel walls and out of those blood vessels. If a forty-two-year-old man has a somewhat high cholesterol, should he be screened yearly with an exercise stress test? Every two years? Every three years? That is just not known.

6. Women suffer from silent ischemia far less often, but they can suffer from it. Indeed, there is some reason to believe that silent ischemia may occur later in life in women but then may occur with greater frequency. However, there seems to be no program for screening women for silent ischemia.

It would, of course, be nice to detect silent ischemia and prevent heart attacks and death in thousands of persons, but the benefits must be weighed against the financial costs and the consequences of working up the many false positives. There is an even more basic question. Suppose we took the high-risk persons without symptoms—those who smoke more than half a pack a day, have an elevated cholesterol or blood pressure—and did no further work-up but merely worked to control the risk factor(s). Would the end result be any different from that obtained from doing stress tests, then more sophisticated work-ups, followed by either medical or surgical treatment when narrowed coronary vessels are found? In other words, would the results be just as good by focusing on the major risk factors and thus avoiding the false positive stress and Holter tests, the dangers of heart catheterization or surgery, and the enormous expense? No one knows the answer to that pivotal question.

We must have more studies and more answers before jumping on the stress test–Holter monitor bandwagon. It is also worth noting that the exercise stress test alone will probably cost more than the entire Health-Full-Life seventeen-point prevention program. Costs like that can bankrupt the health insurance industry—or force them to raise premiums to an unacceptable level.

As for the case cited earlier of the forty-year-old man who had high blood pressure, smoked heavily, and had a high cholesterol, the lawyer said it was malpractice not to do a stress test on this man even though he had no symptoms. That is ridiculous. In our state of knowledge, the doctor should have attempted to lower the cholesterol and blood pressure and persuade the man to stop smoking. That would be a responsible and reasonable approach; the exercise stress test should have been optional.

The controversy over the issue of myocardial ischemia is just beginning. It is likely to heat up substantially in the next few years. For now, I do not recommend a routine work-up for myocardial ischemia for people who have no symptoms.

The program I have proposed is for the healthy adult. It is not physician-intensive. On the other hand, if an individual has persistent symptoms, such as vaginal bleeding or a cough that continues after the patient has stopped smoking, he or she should go to a physician. This program will allow the physician to focus on the symptomatic patient and leave prevention largely to the public and the nurse or paraprofessional.

I want to reemphasize the point about symptoms. If you have continuing symptoms, you are no longer a presumably healthy adult. You may well be perfectly healthy, but you cannot be sure until you have the symptoms analyzed. I have summarized some of the most important symptoms to look for in table 28.

If this program is to succeed, it will have to benefit everyone—the participant, the physician, the employer, and the insurance carrier. I believe it does. Employers are appalled by health costs and are demanding reduction in employee benefits. Unions are desperately trying to protect their health benefits. Both should embrace Health-Full-Life or similar programs—absenteeism would diminish, morale at the workplace would improve, and employees would be healthier. Everyone would benefit.

The program must remain low-cost. Recently, Louise Russell of the Brookings Institute has challenged all of us advocating prevention with a thoughtful monograph entitled *Is Prevention Better Than Cure?* She argues for very careful and thorough cost-effectiveness analyses of prevention activities; a cogent point, since if such activities are not cost-effective, they will not be adopted by the insurance carriers.

TABLE 28

Symptoms That Require Investigation by a Physician

Disease	Symptom
Coronary heart disease, stroke, hypertension	Persistent or recurrent headaches, fainting; extreme shortness of breath after exercise; severe leg pain after exercise; pain over anterior left chest or down left arm after exertion
Bronchitis (chronic)	Chronic cough that persists after stopping smoking
Breast cancer	Nipple retraction; bleeding from nipple; change in breast appearance; pain in breast when not menstruating; dimpling or puckering of skin
Uterine cancer	Vaginal bleeding between periods
Colon cancer	Blood in bowel movements; black, tarry bowel movements (does not apply if taking iron pills); change in size of bowel movements (thin, pencil-like, or ribbonlike)
Anemia	Unexplained and persistent weakness or pallor
Glaucoma	Blurring of vision; eye pain; halos around objects; persistent headache
Diabetes	Unusual thirst; excessive urinating; unexplained weight loss with a good appetite
Thyroid disease	Unusual intolerance of either cold or warm weather; weight loss despite a voracious appetite; unexplained palpitations
Lung cancer or other lung diseases	Persistent cough, spitting up blood, or shortness of breath
Urinary tract infection	Pain on urination or very frequent need to urinate
Prostate tumor or overgrowth	Inability to pass urine normally; blood in urine

Also: look for change in size and color (getting darker) of skin moles or skin sores that will not heal. See a skin specialist immediately.

This table is not meant to be comprehensive. I have included the most frequently reported symptoms for many of the serious diseases afflicting adults.

As I have indicated, cost-effectiveness analyses carried out by biostatisticians in the Department of Preventive Medicine and Community Health at the New Jersey Medical School show clearly that the Health-Full-Life Program works. The program saves companies money, and it saves individuals from the burden of avoidable illness. The cost-effectiveness analysis was very conservative. It included all the costs, but only the benefits from cancer, stroke, and heart disease prevention. The potential benefits from reduction in the severity of automobile accidents, prevention of low back pain, possible prevention of osteoporosis, and possible dietary prevention of certain cancers are harder to calculate and were therefore excluded.

If adults in this country would follow this program, how many years might it add to their lives on the average? If all cancer, stroke, and coronary heart disease were eliminated in the United States, the life expectancy of an adult would increase by eight to ten years. If this program were followed, the coronary heart disease, stroke, and cancer burden would be reduced at least 50 percent, and that should result in an increase in average life expectancy for an adult of four to five years.

The health insurance industry could play an extraordinary role in keeping people healthy by directing their efforts to encouraging compliance with programs such as Health-Full-Life. They could do so in three ways. First, they could undertake far more extensive public education programs that focus on disease prevention. Second, they could pay for Pap smears, mammography, Hemoccult testing, colonoscopy, and the other tests I have suggested. Third, they could tie their premiums to health-promoting activities that are fully documented. Since knowledge of the amount smoked is, for the most part, dependent on self-reporting, I would not favor gearing premiums to the amount allegedly smoked. Similarly, the data would not permit relating premium size to amount of exercise. But premiums could be reduced for those who determine cholesterol and HDL levels, obtain Pap smears, Hemoccults and colonoscopy examination for polyp removal, and then try to correct abnormalities such as a high cholesterol. Fortunately, there is evidence that the health insurance industry is beginning to commit itself to prevention programs like Health-Full-Life, which is very encouraging.

Health insurance carriers should not be allowed to refuse to pay for a program such as Health-Full-Life on the grounds that it would add to premium costs, since they *are* paying for routine X rays, electrocardiograms, unnecessary physical examinations, and useless laboratory studies. If they would stop paying for worthless studies, they would easily be able to pay for much-needed programs such as Health-Full-Life.

I do believe we will need to include financial incentives to entice the American public into taking charge of their own health *before* they develop symptoms or illness. One incentive might be a rebate or dividend of some sort for those who remain enrolled in a Health-Full-Life type of program for five to seven years and who also remain with a given insurance carrier. Or there might be a reduction in the amount a subscriber would pay for subsequent treatment or hospitalization. I would also like to see life and health insurance carriers sequester a small part of the yearly premium in a special account so that an individual who continues coverage starting in early adulthood would accumulate several thousand dollars by age forty; the yearly interest from that small sequestered fund could pay for all future prevention activities.

At present, the American public is just not practicing effective prevention. A Gallup poll taken for the American Cancer Society, and published in February 1984, shows that only 14 percent of men and 10 percent of women over age fifty are having annual tests for intestinal bleeding; only 15 percent of women over the age of fifty have yearly mammographic examinations; half the women examine their breasts for lumps at least three times a year, but only 27 percent do it monthly (and probably half of all these women perform the examination improperly).

The best participation was with the Pap smear; 79 percent of women between twenty and thirty-nine had a Pap smear at least every three years. For women over age forty, the usage was not as good, 57 percent having a Pap smear at least every three years.

A study of breast and cervical cancer screening by Rodney A. Haward, M.D., and his colleagues from the University of California at Los Angeles, published in the May 1988 issue of *Archives of Internal Medicine,* showed that women who were uninsured, in lower socioeconomic groups, or were over age fifty, received inadequate screening for these two important cancers.

Generally, similar results were reported from the National Health Interview Survey of Health Promotion and Disease Prevention in 1985. Only one-third of women examined their breasts at least six times a year, and only half reported a breast examination by a professional in the last year. In that survey, seat belt usage showed the most encouraging results. By the last three months of 1984, 41 percent used belts most of the time.

There is obviously room for much improvement.

If health insurance carriers adopt the Health-Full-Life Program, we will change the face of American medicine and health. At long last the people of this country will act to prevent disease rather than waiting until illness occurs and *then* trying to get it treated. And as an added desirable effect, by practicing prevention, we may be able to gain control of our ever-increasing health costs. It is an idea whose time has come.

Index

About the Author

Donald B. Louria, M.D., trained at Harvard Medical School, Cornell, and the National Institutes of Health. In 1986, he was named Physician of the Year by the American Cancer Society, New Jersey Division. He is the author of four books, including the bestseller *The Drug Scene*, and hundreds of articles for professional journals. Dr. Louria heads a medical school department in Newark, New Jersey, which has the nation's largest AIDS research program.

Additional copies of *Your Healthy Body, Your Healthy Life* may be ordered by sending a check for $12.95 (please add the following for postage and handling: $1.50 for the first copy, $.50 for each added copy) to:

MasterMedia Limited
215 Park Avenue South
Suite 1601
New York, NY 10003
(212) 260-5600

Dr. Louria is available for speeches and workshops. Please contact MasterMedia's Speakers' Bureau for availability and fee arrangements. Call Tony Colao at (201) 359-1612.

Other MasterMedia Books

THE PREGNANCY AND MOTHERHOOD DIARY: Planning the First Year of Your Second Career, by Susan Schiffer Stautberg, is the first and only undated appointment diary that shows how to manage pregnancy and career. ($12.95 spiralbound)

CITIES OF OPPORTUNITY: Finding the Best Place to Work, Live and Prosper in the 1990's and Beyond, by Dr. John Tepper Marlin, explores the job and living options for the next decade and into the next century. This consumer guide and handbook, written by one of the world's experts on cities, selects and features forty-six American cities and metropolitan areas. ($13.95 paper, $24.95 cloth)

THE DOLLARS AND SENSE OF DIVORCE, by Dr. Judith Briles, is the first book to combine practical tips on overcoming the legal hurdles with planning before, during, and after divorce. ($10.95 paper)

OUT THE ORGANIZATION: How Fast Could You Find a New Job?, by Madeleine and Robert Swain, is written for the millions of Americans whose jobs are no longer safe, whose companies are not loyal, and who face futures of uncertainty. It gives advice on finding a new job or starting your own business. ($11.95 paper, $17.95 cloth)

AGING PARENTS AND YOU: A Complete Handbook to Help You Help Your Elders Maintain a Healthy, Productive and

Independent Life, by Eugenia Anderson-Ellis and Marsha Dryan, is a complete guide to providing care to aging relatives. It gives practical advice and resources to the adults who are helping their elders lead productive and independent lives. ($9.95 paper)

CRITICISM IN YOUR LIFE: How to Give It, How to Take It, How to Make It Work for You, by Dr. Deborah Bright, offers practical advice, in an upbeat, readable, and realistic fashion, for turning criticism into control. Charts and diagrams guide the reader into managing criticism from bosses, spouses, relationships, children, friends, neighbors, and in-laws. ($17.95 cloth)

BEYOND SUCCESS: How Volunteer Service Can Help You Begin Making a Life Instead of Just a Living, by John F. Raynolds III and Eleanor Raynolds, C.B.E., is a unique how-to book targeted to business and professional people considering volunteer work, senior citizens who wish to fill leisure time meaningfully, and students trying out various career options. The book is filled with interviews with celebrities, CEOs, and average citizens who talk about the benefits of service work. ($9.95 paper, $19.95 cloth)

MANAGING IT ALL: Time-Saving Ideas for Career, Family Relationships, and Self, by Beverly Benz Treuille and Susan Schiffer Stautberg, is written for women who are juggling careers and families. Over two hundred career women (ranging from a TV anchorwoman to an investment banker) were interviewed. The book contains many humorous anecdotes on saving time and improving the quality of life for self and family. ($9.95 paper)

REAL LIFE 101: (Almost) Surviving Your First Year Out of College, by Susan Kleinman, supplies welcome advice to those facing "real life" for the first time, focusing on work, money, health, and how to deal with freedom and responsibility. ($9.95 paper)

Keep current about health promotion and disease prevention with *THE HEALTH-FULL-LIFE NEWSLETTER*—an exciting new bimonthly publication.

A joint venture of Health-Full-Life Inc. and the Department of Preventive Medicine of the New Jersey Medical School.

There is nothing quite like it. We tell you what is new and what is important for your health.

For more information, contact:

Mr. Michael Powers
M. J. Powers & Co. Publishers
374 Milburn Avenue
Milburn, NJ 07041
(201) 467-4556